PAIN MEDICINE
A CASE-BASED LEARNING SERIES

The Spine

Other books in this series:

 The Shoulder and Elbow
9780323758772

 The Hip and Pelvis
9780323762977

 The Knee
9780323762588

 Headache and Facial Pain
9780323834568

 The Wrist and Hand
9780323834537

 The Chest Wall and Abdomen
9780323846882

 The Ankle and Foot
9780323870382

PAIN MEDICINE
A CASE-BASED
LEARNING SERIES

The Spine

STEVEN D. WALDMAN, MD, JD

ELSEVIER

Elsevier
1600 John F. Kennedy Blvd.
Ste 1800
Philadelphia, PA 19103-2899

PAIN MEDICINE: A CASE-BASED LEARNING SERIES ISBN: 978-0-323-75636-5
THE SPINE

Notice

Practitioners and researchers must always rely on their own experience and knowledge in evaluating and using any information, methods, compounds or experiments described herein. Because of rapid advances in the medical sciences, in particular, independent verification of diagnoses and drug dosages should be made. To the fullest extent of the law, no responsibility is assumed by Elsevier, authors, editors or contributors for any injury and/or damage to persons or property as a matter of products liability, negligence or otherwise, or from any use or operation of any methods, products, instructions, or ideas contained in the material herein.

Library of Congress Control Number: 2020950564

Executive Content Strategist: Michael Houston
Content Development Specialist: Jeannine Carrado/Laura Klien
Director, Content Development: Ellen Wurm-Cutter
Publishing Services Manager: Shereen Jameel
Senior Project Manager: Karthikeyan Murthy
Design Direction: Amy Buxton

Printed in India

Last digit is the print number: 9 8 7 6 5 4 3 2

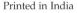
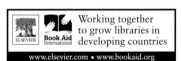

Working together
to grow libraries in
developing countries

www.elsevier.com • www.bookaid.org

To Peanut and David H.
SDW

"When you go after honey with a balloon, the great thing is to not let the bees know you're coming."
WINNIE THE POOH

It's Harder Than It Looks
MAKING THE CASE FOR CASE-BASED LEARNING

For sake of full disclosure, I was one of those guys. You know, the ones who wax poetic about how hard it is to teach our students how to do procedures. Let me tell you, teaching folks how to do epidurals on women in labor certainly takes its toll on the coronary arteries. It's true, I am amazing. . .I am great. . .I have nerves of steel. Yes, I could go on like this for hours. . .but you have heard it all before. But, it's again that time of year when our new students sit eagerly before us, full of hope and dreams. . .and that harsh reality comes slamming home. . .it is a lot harder to teach beginning medical students "doctoring" than it looks.

A few years ago, I was asked to teach first-year medical and physician assistant students how to take a history and perform a basic physical exam. In my mind I thought "this should be easy. . .no big deal". I won't have to do much more than show up. After all, I was the guy who wrote that amazing book on physical diagnosis. After all, I had been teaching medical students, residents, and fellows how to do highly technical (and dangerous, I might add) interventional pain management procedures since right after the Civil War. Seriously, it was no big deal...I could do it in my sleep. . .with one arm tied behind my back. . .blah. . .blah. . .blah.

For those of you who have had the privilege of teaching "doctoring," you already know what I am going to say next. *It's harder than it looks!* Let me repeat this to disabuse any of you who, like me, didn't get it the first time. *It is harder than it looks!* I only had to meet with my first-year medical and physician assistant students a couple of times to get it through my thick skull: **It really is harder than it looks**. In case you are wondering, the reason that our students look back at us with those blank, confused, bored, and ultimately dismissive looks is simple: They lack context. That's right, they lack the context to understand what we are talking about.

It's really that simple. . .or hard. . .depending on your point of view or stubbornness, as the case may be. To understand why context is king, you have to look only as far as something as basic as the Review of Systems. The Review of Systems is about as basic as it gets, yet why is it so perplexing to our students? Context. I guess it should come as no surprise to anyone that the student is completely lost when you talk about. . .let's say. . .the "constitutional" portion of the Review of Systems, without the context of what a specific constitutional finding, say a fever or chills, might mean to a patient who is suffering from the acute onset of headaches. If you tell the student that you need to ask about fever, chills, and the other "constitutional" stuff and you take it no further, you might as well be talking about the

International Space Station. Just save your breath; it makes absolutely no sense to your students. Yes, they want to please, so they will memorize the elements of the Review of Systems, but that is about as far as it goes. On the other hand, if you present the case of Jannette Patton, a 28-year-old first-year medical resident with a fever and headache, you can see the lights start to come on. By the way, this is what Jannette looks like, and as you can see, Jannette is sicker than a dog. This, at its most basic level, is what *Case-Based Learning* is all about.

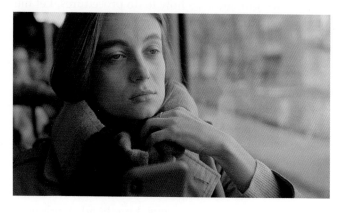

I would like to tell you that, smart guy that I am, I immediately saw the light and became a convert to *Case-Based Learning*. But truth be told, it was COVID-19 that really got me thinking about *Case-Based Learning*. Before the COVID-19 pandemic, I could just drag the students down to the med/surg wards and walk into a patient room and riff. Everyone was a winner. For the most part, the patients loved to play along and thought it was cool. The patient and the bedside was all I needed to provide the context that was necessary to illustrate what I was trying to teach—the why headache and fever don't mix kind of stuff. Had COVID-19 not rudely disrupted my ability to teach at the bedside, I suspect that you would not be reading this *Preface*, as I would not have had to write it. Within a very few days after the COVID-19 pandemic hit, my days of bedside teaching disappeared, but my students still needed context. This got me focused on how to provide the context they needed. The answer was, of course, *Case-Based Learning*. What started as a desire to provide context. . .because it really was **harder than it looked**. . .led me to begin work on this eight-volume *Case-Based Learning* textbook series. What you will find within these volumes are a bunch of fun, real-life cases that help make each patient come alive for the student. These cases provide the contextual teaching points that make it easy for the teacher to explain why, when Jannette's chief complaint is, *"My head is killing me and I've got a fever,"* it is a big deal.

Have fun!

Steven D. Waldman, MD, JD
Spring 2021

ACKNOWLEDGMENTS

A very special thanks to my editors, Michael Houston, PhD, Jeannine Carrado, and Karthikeyan Murthy, for all of their hard work and perseverance in the face of disaster. Great editors such as Michael, Jeannine, and Karthikeyan make their authors look great, for they not only understand how to bring the Three Cs of great writing...Clarity + Consistency + Conciseness...to the author's work, but unlike me, they can actually punctuate and spell!

Steven D. Waldman, MD, JD

P.S. ...Sorry for all the ellipses, guys!

CONTENTS

VIDEO CONTENTS

Mimi Braverman

A 68-Year-Old Female With Acute Worsening Neck and Occipital Pain

LEARNING OBJECTIVES

- Learn how rheumatoid arthritis affects the cervical spine.
- Develop a high index of suspicion for the potential for life-threatening complications of unrecognized rheumatoid arthritis-induced atlantoaxial instability.
- Learn to identify risk factors associated with an increased incidence of rheumatoid arthritis affecting the cervical spine.
- Learn the clinical presentation of atlantoaxial instability secondary to rheumatoid arthritis.
- Learn the classic clinical presentation of rheumatoid arthritis affecting the hands.
- Understand the role of laboratory testing and imaging in the evaluation of rheumatoid arthritis-induced atlantoaxial instability.
- Learn to identify the neurologic findings associated with cervical myelopathy.
- Develop an understanding of the role of disease-modifying drugs in the prevention of rheumatoid arthritis-induced damage to the cervical spine.

Mimi Braverman

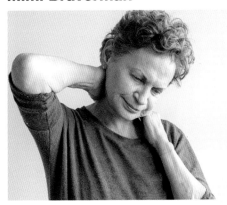

Mimi Braverman is a 68-year-old female with the chief complaint of, "I know that you will think I'm crazy, but it feels like my head is going to fall off." Mrs. Braverman said that she knew "something wasn't right with her head" for several months. She had attributed the head and neck discomfort to "old age" and she chose to "just live with the pain." An avid knitter, it wasn't until a couple of weeks ago, when she looked down at her knitting, that she felt and heard a "clunk" in her neck. The patient noted that the "clunk" really scared her and she was worried that "something was really wrong." She said that the "clunk" happened a couple of more times and it scared her so much that now she was afraid to knit...even though the occupational therapist told her that "knitting was good for her hands."

When the patient was asked to use one finger to point to the area where the "clunk" came from, she pointed to the posterior occiput. The patient noted that when she looked down, pain shot up into the back of her head as well as into her face and ear. She also noted that she felt sudden electric shocks that went from the back of her head down into her arms. The pain went away as soon as she raised her head. When asked to describe the character of the pain, the patient stated that the pain in the back of her head felt like when your leg goes to sleep, a kind of pins and needles sensation. She noted that the pain down her arms was different...that it was like an electric shock. When asked what made her pain worse, she stated emphatically that it only occurred when she looked down. When asked what made her pain better, she said, "looking up." The patient rated her pain as a 5 on a 1 to 10 verbal analogue scale with 10 being the worst and 1 being the mildest.

When asked about associated symptoms, Mrs. Braverman noted that since she began having the "clunking" sensation, that she was also "losing urine" and had had several accidents when she didn't make it to the bathroom. When questioned, she admitted that she noticed that her bottom was numb when she wiped after going to the bathroom.

On physical examination, the patient was normotensive and afebrile. Her cognition was normal, as was her nutritional status. Bilateral cataracts were noted in both of her eyes. Her cardiopulmonary examination was unremarkable, as was her abdominal examination There was no peripheral edema.

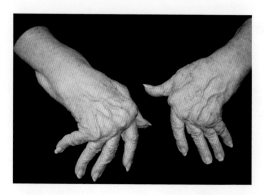

Fig. 1.1 Ulnar drift. (From Chung KC, Pushman AG. Current concepts in the management of the rheumatoid hand. *J Hand Surg.* 2011;36(4):736—747, Fig. 4.)

Examination of the hands revealed severe ulnar drift bilaterally (Fig. 1.1). No active synovitis was noted. Examination of her feet revealed severe arthritis. Careful examination of the cervical spine revealed crepitus with flexion. At about 30 degrees of flexion, an audible and palpable clunk was appreciated. This clunk elicited a positive Lhermitte's sign. When the cervical spine was returned to the neutral position, the patient noted that the shocklike pain completely disappeared.

The patient's neurologic examination revealed that the patient had an unsteady gait. Examination of the deep tendon reflexes of the upper and lower extremities revealed hyperreflexia throughout. Babinski sign was present, as was Hoffman's sign (Videos 1.1 and 1.2 on Expert Consult). Clonus was not present. Sensory examination revealed no evidence of peripheral or entrapment neuropathy, but there was decreased rectal sphincter tone and perineal numbness.

Key Clinical Points—What's Important and What's Not

THE HISTORY

- Chief complaint of "it feels like my head is going to fall off"
- Recent onset of a "clunking" sensation and sound in Mimi's upper cervical spine
- Pins and needles-like pain in posterior occiput
- Electric shocklike pain radiating down upper extremities bilaterally
- Short duration of symptoms associated with flexion of cervical spine
- Symptoms triggered by flexion of cervical spine
- Symptoms relieved by returning cervical spine to neutral position
- Urinary and fecal incontinence
- Perineal numbness
- Hand clumsiness

THE PHYSICAL EXAMINATION

- The patient is scared and upset
- Patient thought she had cancer
- Bilateral hand deformities—ulnar drift (see Fig. 1.1)
- Decreased range of motion of affected joints
- Bilateral foot deformities
- Decreased range of motion of wrist and fingers
- Crepitus on flexion of cervical spine
- Sudden palpable and audible "clunk" with flexion of the cervical spine
- Elicitation of Lhermitte's sign with flexion of the cervical spine
- Unsteady gait
- Hyperreflexic deep tendon reflexes throughout
- Babinski sign present (see Video 1.1 on Expert Consult)
- Hoffman sign present (see Video 1.2 on Expert Consult)
- Perineal numbness
- Decreased sphincter tone

OTHER FINDINGS OF NOTE

- Bilateral cataracts
- Normal cardiovascular examination
- Normal pulmonary examination
- Normal abdominal examination
- No peripheral edema

 What Tests Would You Order?

The following tests were ordered:
- Rheumatoid factor and anticitrullinated protein antibody titers
- Plain flexion and extension radiographs of the cervical spine with open mouth views to evaluate the odontoid. I asked that the radiology technician use great care when flexing and extending the cervical spine.
- Computed tomography (CT) scan of the cervical spine to document precisely the relative position of the odontoid relative to the foramen magnum and to identify the presence of other bony abnormalities, including subaxial subluxation, that might be contributing to the neurologic symptoms. I also hoped to define better what was causing compromise of the subarachnoid space.
- Magnetic resonance imaging (MRI) of the cervical spine to identify retro-odontoid pseudotumor that might be compromising the cervical spinal cord. I also wanted to try and evaluate the condition of the transverse ligament and identify any edema and/or erosion of the odontoid process,

as well as identify any of the joints. I also hoped to ascertain the appearance of the cervical spinal cord.

- Somatosensory-evoked potentials to quantify the presence and extent of cervical myelopathy

TEST RESULTS

As expected, Mimi's rheumatoid factor and anticitrullinated protein antibody titers were markedly elevated, confirming my clinical diagnosis of rheumatoid arthritis. Given the duration and extent of Mimi's disease, it was not surprising that all of her imaging results were markedly abnormal. Flexion and extension cervical spine radiographs revealed significant anterior subluxation of C1 on C2 with an anterior atlantodental interval of 5 mm. There was extensive subaxial disease with subluxation of C3 on C4 and disc space narrowing, anterior osteophytosis, and facet joint disease of the lower cervical spine (Fig. 1.2). Her CT scan revealed atlantoaxial dislocation and cervical kyphosis (Fig. 1.3). MRI scan of the cervical spine revealed atlantoaxial instability with proximal migration of the odontoid process and severe spinal cord compression at C3-C4. The spinal cord draped over the odontoid process (Fig. 1.4). Somatosensory-evoked potentials were consistent with significant cervical myelopathy (Fig. 1.5).

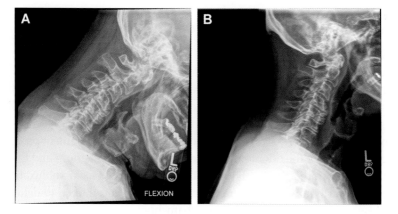

Fig. 1.2 Plain lateral radiographs of the cervical spine in flexion (A) and extension (B) reveal significant anterior subluxation of C1 on C2 with an anterior atlantodental interval of 5 mm. There is extensive subaxial disease with subluxation of C3 on C4 and disc space narrowing, anterior osteophytosis, and facet joint disease of the lower cervical spine. (From DeQuattro K, Imboden JB. Neurologic manifestations of rheumatoid arthritis. *Rheum Dis Clin North Am.* 2017;43(4):561–571, Fig. 1.)

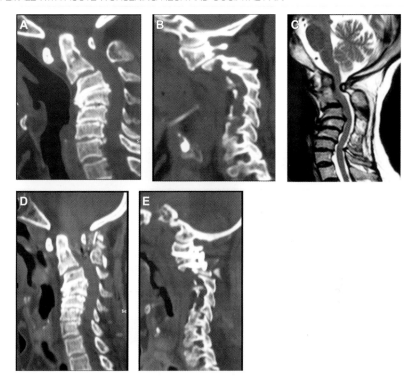

Fig. 1.3 Computed tomography (CT) scan of the cervical spine in an elderly female. (A) Sagittal image of CT scan showing atlantoaxial dislocation and cervical kyphosis. (B) Sagittal CT scan with cut passing through the facets. It shows type 1 atlantoaxial facetal dislocation. (From Goel A, Kaswa A, Shah A. Role of atlantoaxial and subaxial spinal instability in pathogenesis of spinal "degeneration"—related cervical kyphosis. *World Neurosurg*. 2017;101:702–709, Fig. 1A & B.)

 Clinical Correlation—Putting It All Together

What is the diagnosis?
- Atlantoaxial instability secondary to rheumatoid arthritis involving the cervical spine

The Science Behind the Diagnosis

The exact pathophysiology of rheumatoid arthritis remains elusive, but recent research that has led to the development of newer disease-modifying agents suggests that abnormal antigens produced by synovial cells elicit the production of multiple autoantibodies. The most important of these autoantibodies appears to be rheumatoid factor and anticitrullinated protein antibodies. Some investigators believe that these antiautoantibodies may act synergistically to cause the joint and organ system damage associated with rheumatoid arthritis (Fig. 1.6).

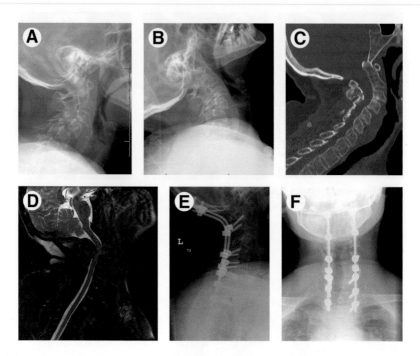

Fig. 1.4 Treatment of combined deformity: AI and subaxial instability. This 39-year-old woman with RA had advanced involvement of the cervical spine with AI and subaxial instability that led to rapid progressive myelopathy with quadriparesis. (A) Flexion and (B) extension views demonstrate subaxial instability at C4 and C5. (C) AI is shown more clearly, with proximal migration of the odontoid process. (D) An MRI T2 sagittal view, depicting severe cord compression at C3-C4 with the cord draped over the odontoid process. This patient was treated with an occiput to T2 fusion with C2-C6 laminectomy (E, lateral view; F, anteroposterior view). She recovered enough strength in her upper and lower extremities to be able to walk 30 feet with a walker. (From Hohl JB, Grabowski G, Donaldson WF. Cervical deformity in rheumatoid arthritis. *Semin Spine Surg.* 2011;23(3):181–187, Fig. 3C & D.)

Approximately 80% of patients suffering from rheumatoid arthritis will have involvement of the cervical spine. Risk factors for cervical spine involvement, which are listed in Box 1.1, include female gender, presence of markers indicating higher disease activity, long duration of disease, delay in use of disease-modifying drugs, and younger age at disease onset. The clinical significance of this involvement can range from asymptomatic to life threatening. Although rheumatoid arthritis has the potential to affect all elements of the cervical spine, the atlantoaxial joint (C1-C2) is most commonly affected (Figs. 1.7, 1.8, and 1.9). If the patient's rheumatoid arthritis is poorly managed, inflammatory destruction of the joint, transverse ligament, and erosion of the odontoid process may occur with resultant atlantoaxial joint instability (Figs. 1.10 and 1.11). Rheumatoid arthritis-induced retro-odontoid pseudotumor formation can exacerbate compression of the cervical spinal cord at this level by causing direct compression of the spinal cord and by weakening the transverse and alar ligaments,

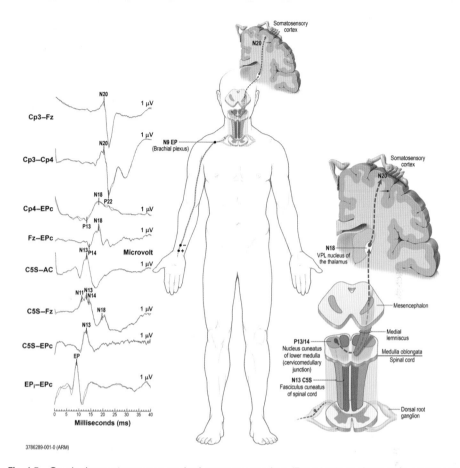

Fig. 1.5 Cervical somatosensory-evoked response testing. (From Levin K, Chauvel P. *Handbook of Clinical Neurology*. Vol. 160. Amsterdam: Elsevier; 2019: Fig. 35.1.)

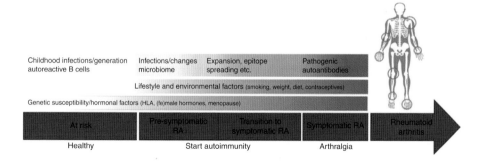

Fig. 1.6 Overview of the factors that may contribute to the development of rheumatoid arthritis. (From van Delft MAM, Huizinga WJ. An overview of autoantibodies in rheumatoid arthritis. *J Autoimmun.* 2020;110.)

BOX 1.1 ■ Risk Factors for Cervical Spine Involvement in Rheumatoid Arthritis

- Female gender
- Presence of markers indicating higher disease activity
  - Positive rheumatoid factor
  - Significantly elevated erythrocyte sedimentation rate
  - High C-reactive protein level
  - High disease activity score
- Long duration of disease
- Delay in use of disease-modifying agents
- Younger age at disease onset

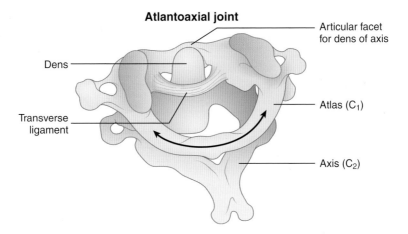

Fig. 1.7 Anatomy of the atlantoaxial joint.

causing additional C1-C2 instability (Figs. 1.12 and 1.13). If the C1-C2 instability worsens, the odontoid process may migrate superiorly and impinge on the medulla and spinal cord (Fig. 1.14). Complicating the clinical picture is the fact that other rheumatoid arthritis-induced cervical spine abnormalities, including subaxial subluxation and facet joint abnormalities, may contribute to the patient's symptoms (see Figs. 1.4 and 1.5).

The physical finding of ulnar drift is pathognomonic for rheumatoid arthritis (see Fig. 1.1). Ulnar drift is the term of art used to describe two separate rheumatoid arthritis-induced changes of the metacarpophalangeal joint: (1) ulnar rotation and (2) ulnar shift (Fig. 1.15). Ulnar rotation is the result of rotation of the proximal phalanx in the ulnar axis relative to the metacarpal head. Ulnar shift is the result of ulnar translation of the base of the proximal phalanx relative to the metacarpal heads (see Fig. 1.15).

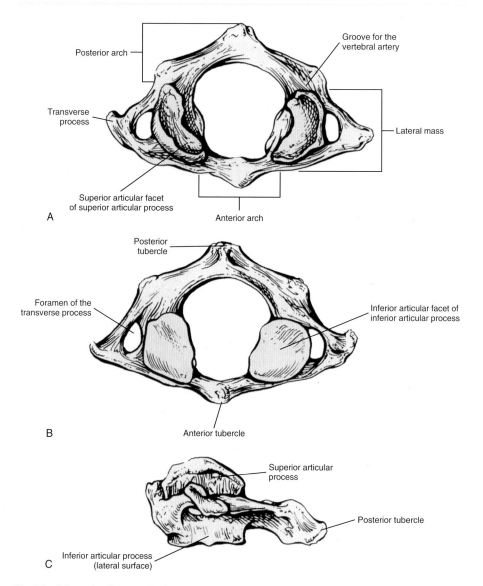

Fig. 1.8 Atlas—the first cervical vertebra. Superior (A), inferior (B), and, lateral (C) views of the first cervical vertebra—the atlas. Superior (D), inferior (E), and, lateral (F) views of the first cervical vertebra—the atlas. (G) Close-up (superior view) of the lateral mass of the atlas. Notice the colliculus atlantis and sulcus (foveola) on the medial surface of the lateral mass. (From Cramer G, Darby S. *Clinical Anatomy of the Spine, Spinal Cord and ANS*. 3rd ed. St. Louis: Mosby; 2014:135–209.)

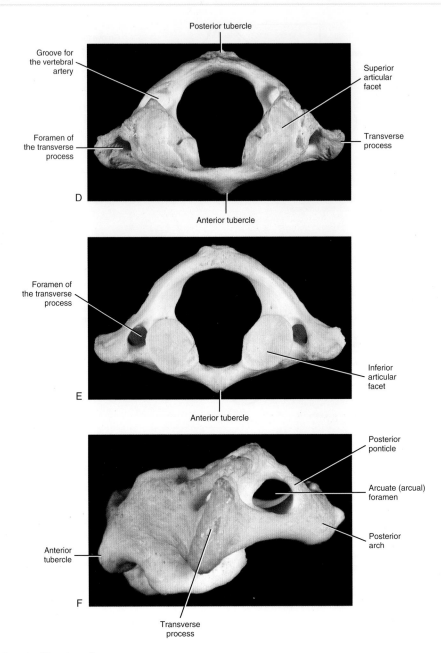

Fig. 1.8   (Continued).

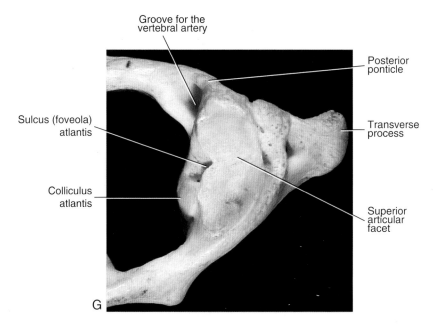

Fig. 1.8   (Continued).

MANAGEMENT AND TREATMENT

Once the damage caused to the atlantoaxial joint has occurred, there is no effective medication management. Corticosteroids may provide some short-term symptomatic relief, but there is no evidence that they can prevent progression of neurologic deficits over the long term. The use of physical modalities may help provide symptomatic relief. A soft cervical collar may help limit flexion of the cervical spine. Local heat may provide relief of muscle spasms. Ice packs may also provide symptomatic relief of localized pain and muscle spasm.

Once atlantoaxial instability secondary to rheumatoid arthritis-induced damage to the cervical spine has occurred, surgical stabilization is indicated. Studies have shown that surgical stabilization not only improves quality of life and function, but also increases life expectancy in this patient population. Surgical options available for the treatment of atlantoaxial instability include (1) posterior transarticular screws, (2) posterior sublaminar wiring, (3) Halifax clamping, and (4) screw-rod constructs (Fig. 1.16). The choice of surgical

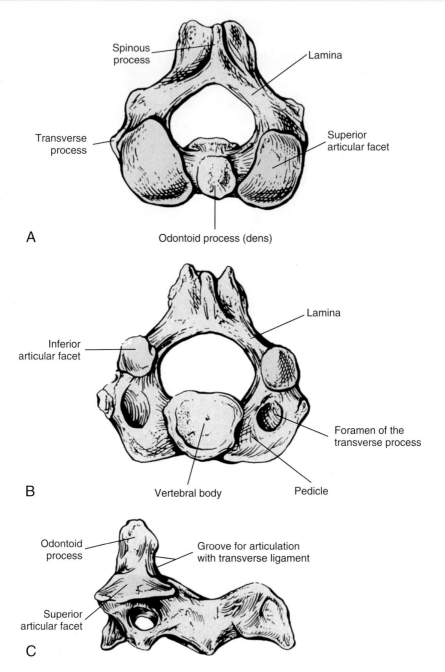

Fig. 1.9 Axis—the second cervical vertebra. Superior (A), inferior (B), and, lateral (C) views of the second cervical vertebra—the axis. Superior (D), inferior (E), and, lateral (F) views of the second cervical vertebra—the axis. (G) Anterior-posterior "open mouth" view of the upper cervical region showing the atlas, axis, and related bony structures. (From Cramer G, Darby S. *Clinical Anatomy of the Spine, Spinal Cord and ANS*. 3rd ed. St. Louis: Mosby; 2014.)

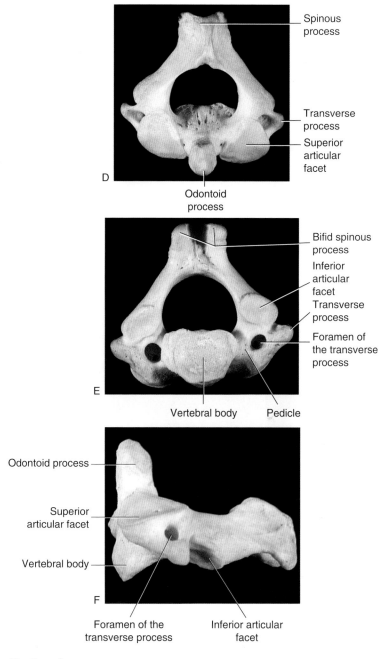

Spinous process

Transverse process

Superior articular facet

D

Odontoid process

Bifid spinous process

Inferior articular facet

Transverse process

Foramen of the transverse process

E

Vertebral body   Pedicle

Odontoid process

Superior articular facet

Vertebral body

F

Foramen of the transverse process

Inferior articular facet

Fig. 1.9 (Continued).

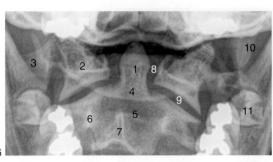

1. Odontoid process (dens)
2. C1 Lateral mass
3. C1 Transverse process
4. C1 Posterior arch
5. C2 Vertebral body
6. C2 Pedicle
7. C2 Spinous process
8. Odontoid-lateral mass space
9. Lateral atlanto-axial articulation
10. Styloid process
11. Unerupted third molar

Fig. 1.9 (Continued).

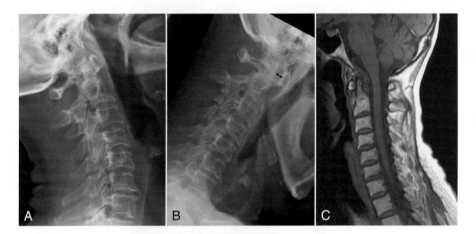

Fig. 1.10 (A) Lateral radiograph of the cervical spine in extension shows normal C1-C2 alignment. (B) On cervical flexion, however, there is widening of the predental space owing to C1-C2 instability (*double-headed arrow*). (C) The sagittal T1-weighted magnetic resonance image shows erosion of the dorsal aspect of the odontoid peg. (From Waldman SD, Campbell RSD. *Imaging of Pain*. Philadelphia: Saunders; 2011: Fig 24.1.)

technique will be driven by the experience of the operator as well as the quality of vertebral bone as corticosteroid-induced osteoporosis is often present. Other factors affecting the choice of surgical technique include coexistent sub-axial and atlanto-occipital instability.

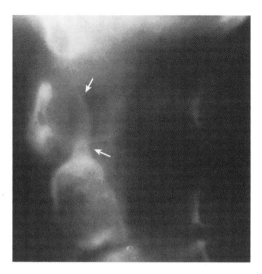

Fig. 1.11 Abnormalities of the cervical spine: odontoid process erosions. Lateral conventional tomogram reveals severe destruction of the odontoid process *(arrows)*, which has been reduced to an irregular, pointed protuberance. (From Resnick D, Kransdorf MJ. *Bone and Joint Imaging*. 3rd ed. Philadelphia: Saunders; 2004: 244.)

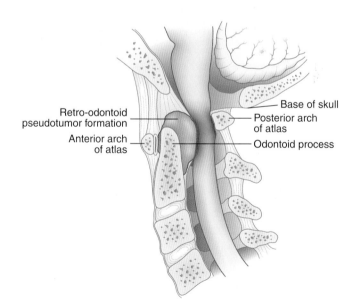

Fig. 1.12 Rheumatoid arthritis-induced retro-odontoid pseudotumor formation can exacerbate compression of the cervical spinal cord at this level by direct compression of the spinal cord and by weakening the transverse and alar ligaments, causing additional C1-C2 instability.

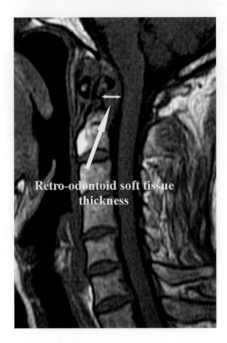

Fig. 1.13 Midsagittal T1-weighted magnetic resonance imaging showing presence of retro-odontoid soft tissue. (From Ryu J II, Han MH, Cheong JH, et al. The effects of clinical factors and retro-odontoid soft tissue thickness on atlantoaxial instability in patients with rheumatoid arthritis. *World Neurosurg*. 2017;103:364–370, Fig. 2.)

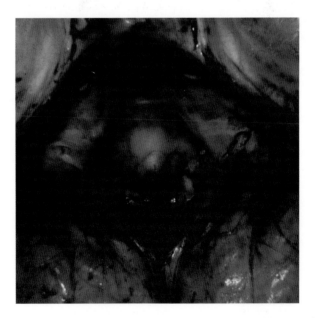

Fig. 1.14 Gross anatomic specimen of the base of the skull of a patient with severe rhematoid arthritis. Looking down into the foramen magnum from above, a bony protuberance can be seen. This upward dislocation of the odontoid process of the axis pushes the medulla and spinal cord backward. (From Kovacs G, Alafuzoff I. *Handbook of Clinical Neurology*. Vol. 145. Amsterdam: Elsevier; 2017: Fig. 29.9.)

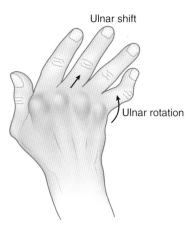

Fig. 1.15 Ulnar drift is the term of art used to describe two separate rheumatoid arthritis-induced changes of the metocarpalphalangeal joint: ulnar rotation ulnar shift.

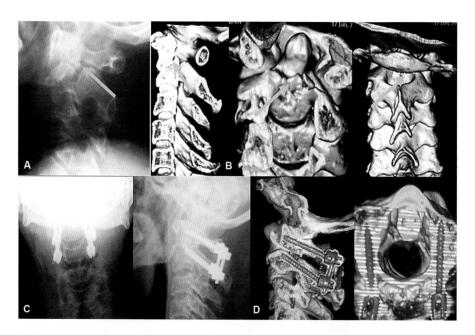

Fig. 1.16 Imaging results of a 34-year-old woman diagnosed with odontoid fracture combined with atlantoaxial dislocation. (A, B) Preoperative sagittal plain radiographs and CT scans showed odontoid fracture with atlantoaxial dislocation. (C) Postoperative anteroposterior and lateral radiograph showing satisfactory restoration of vertebral alignment. (D) On a lateral and axial CT scans 12 months after operation, bone fusion was observed, and fixation remained satisfactory. (From Zheng Y, Hao D, Wang B, He B, Hu H, Zhang H: Clinical outcome of posterior C1−C2 pedicle screw fixation and fusion for atlantoaxial instability: a retrospective study of 86 patients. *J Clin Neurosci.* 2016;32:47−50, Fig. 1.)

HIGH-YIELD TAKEAWAYS

- Prevention of rheumatoid arthritis-induced damage to the cervical spine is highly desirable.
- The early use of conventional, targeted, and biologic disease-modifying drugs is critical to avoid rheumatoid arthritis-induced damage to the cervical spine and resultant atlantoaxial instability. (See Boxes 1.2, 1.3, and 1.4.)
- The diagnosis of atlantoaxial instability should be considered in all patients with rheumatoid arthritis; a high index of suspicion is crucial to avoid disastrous neurologic sequelae and sudden death.
- Early identification of neurologic signs and symptoms associated with atlantoaxial instability is crucial to avoid permanent neurologic damage.
- Surgical stabilization is the treatment of choice for rheumatoid arthritis-induced atlantoaxial instability.

BOX 1.2 ■ Conventional Synthetic Disease-Modifying Antirheumatic Drugs (csDMARDs)

- Auranofin
- Azathioprine
- Cyclophosphamide
- Cyclosporine
- Gold sodium thiomalate
- Hydroxychloroquine sulfate
- Leflunomide
- Methotrexate
- Minocycline
- Mycophenolate
- Sulfasalazine

BOX 1.3 ■ Targeted Synthetic Disease-Modifying Antirheumatic Drugs (tsDMARDs)—Small Molecule Inhibitor

- Xeljanz (tofacitinib)
- Olumiant (baricitinib)

BOX 1.4 ■ Biologic Disease-Modifying Antirheumatic Drugs (bDMARDs)—Biologics

Tumor Necrosis Factor Inhibitors
- Humira (adalimumab)
- Enbrel (etanercept)
- Cimzia (certolizumab pegol)
- Inflectra (infliximab-dyyb)
- Renflexis (infliximab-abda)
- Remicade (infliximab)
- Simponi/Simponi AIRA (golimumab)

Nontumor Necrosis Factor Inhibitors
- Actemra (tocilizumab)
- Orencia (abatecept)
- Rituxan (rituximab)
- Kineret (anakinra)
- Kevzara (sarilumab)

Suggested Readings

Akhavani MA, Paleolog EM, Kang N. Muscle hypoxia in rheumatoid hands: does it play a role in ulnar drift? *J Hand Surg.* 2011;36(4):677−685.

DeQuattro K, Imboden JB. Neurologic manifestation of rheumatoid arthritis. *Rheum Dis Clin North Am.* 2017;43(4):561−571.

Gandhi JS. The rheumatoid hands of Renoir. *Am J Med.* 2019;132(5):658−659.

Gandhi JS, Lee J-Y, Im S-B, Jeong J-H. Use of a C1-C2 facet spacer to treat atlantoaxial instability and basilar invagination associated with rheumatoid arthritis. *World Neurosurg.* 2017;874e13−874e16.

Ryu JI, Han MH, Cheong JH, et al. The effects of clinical factors and retro-odontoid soft tissue thickness on atlantoaxial instability in patients with rheumatoid arthritis. *World Neurosurg.* 2017;103:364−370.

Wu F, Talwalkar S. Surgical management of the rheumatoid hand and wrist. *Orthop Trauma.* 2019;33(1):23−29.

Alex Searcy

A 58-Year-Old Female With Acute Neck Pain

- Learn the common causes of cervical strain.
- Learn the clinical presentation of cervical strain.
- Learn to distinguish cervical strain from cervical radiculopathy.
- Learn the anatomic structures affected by cervical strain.
- Develop an understanding of the treatment options for cervical strain.
- Develop an understanding of the role of interventional pain management in the treatment of cervical strain.

Alex Searcy

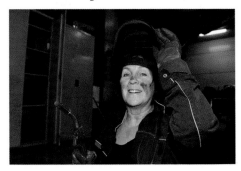

Alex Searcy is a 52-year-old woman with the chief complaint of, "My neck is killing me." I asked her when the pain started and she told me that for the past two weeks, she had been welding girders below the Buck O'Neil bridge. This required her to climb down below the deck of the bridge and stand on a scaffold suspended above the river, which ran about 400 feet beneath the bridge. In order to weld the girders, Alex had to spend her day looking up at the bottom of the bridge, holding her arms above her head to reach the girders. She had been doing this eight hours a day for the past two weeks. Her pain began to come on after about three days on the job. She said, "Doctor, you know I am tough as steel, but this is really bad." When I asked her to show me where the pain was, she rubbed the back of her neck and upper shoulders. I then asked if the pain went into her arms and she said no. . .the pain was just in the neck and shoulders. She denied any numbness, tingling, or weakness in her arms or hands, but noted she had a headache in the back of her head for days and that her neck muscles "felt tight."

Alex described the pain as a "deep, dull ache that worsened when extending her neck to look up at the bottom of the bridge." She told me that this time, "in spite of the neck pain," she kept working as she didn't want the "bridge to fall into the river." Alex went on to say that "it would take a lot more than this neck problem" to make her stay home. She went on to say that it was really not the pain that made her come to see me; it was because she was so tired from having to sleep in a chair at night. She then gave me a crooked smile and said that she "really didn't want to fall asleep while working underneath the Buck O'Neil bridge and then fall off the bridge into the Missouri River." I laughed and agreed with her that that wasn't a good idea. I asked her what she had been doing to manage the pain and she said she had tried over-the-counter Advil and a heating pad, but to no avail. "No oxy for me," she proudly said. . .that was for sissies, and besides, her company did random drug screens.

On physical examination, Alex was afebrile and normotensive. Her head, ears, eyes, nose, and throat (HEENT) examination, including a careful fundoscopic examination, was normal, as was her cardiopulmonary examination. Her abdominal examination revealed a well-healed appendectomy scar and no abnormal mass or organomegaly. There was no peripheral edema. Examination of the neck revealed that Alex was sitting with her head held forward with her neck held stiffly and the shoulders rounded. Palpation of the posterior neck muscles revealed tenderness to deep palpation bilaterally. There was a suggestion of muscle spasm and muscle tightness. Decreased active and passive range of motion was noted. The Spurling test was negative (Fig. 2.1). Alex's neurologic examination was normal; specifically, her upper and lower extremity deep tendon reflexes were physiologic and there was no sensory deficit or weakness. No pathologic reflexes or clonus were identified. Alex denied bowel and bladder symptoms associated with her pain.

I ordered a cervical spine radiograph. Given her physical examination and the lack of antecedent cervical spine trauma (e.g., whiplash injury, fall), I decided to wait on ordering magnetic resonance imaging (MRI) of her cervical spine.

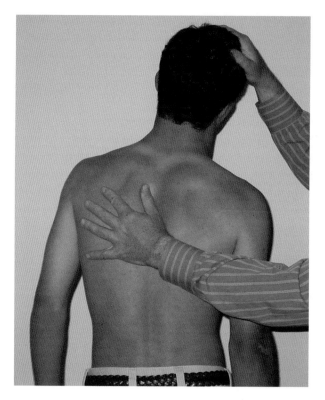

Fig. 2.1 The Spurling test. The Spurling test is performed by extending the neck and then tilting the neck to the painful side. The test is positive if it elicits radicular pain. (From Waldman SD. *Physical Diagnosis of Pain: An Atlas of Signs and Symptoms*. 3rd ed. St. Louis: Elsevier; 2016: Fig. 13.1.)

Key Clinical Points—What's Important and What's Not

THE HISTORY

- Chief complaint: "my neck is killing me"
- Significant sleep disturbance associated with pain
- Recent history of prolonged cervical spine extension while holding her arms above the head while working as a welder
- Lack of other antecedent trauma to head or neck
- Neck stiffness and tightness
- Posterior headache
- No pain radiation into upper extremities
- No numbness or weakness of upper extremities
- Symptoms triggered by flexion and extension of the cervical spine
- No urinary and fecal incontinence
- No pathologic reflexes

THE PHYSICAL EXAMINATION

- The patient is afebrile
- Neck posturing in an attempt to splint neck
- Shoulder rounding to protect and splint neck
- Normal deep tendon reflexes
- Normal upper and lower extremity motor and sensory examination
- No pathologic reflexes
- No clonus
- Negative Spurling sign

OTHER FINDINGS OF NOTE

- Normal cardiovascular examination
- Normal pulmonary examination
- Normal abdominal examination
- No peripheral edema

What Tests Would You Order?

The following tests were ordered:
- Cervical spine radiographs. Given her physical examination and the lack of antecedent cervical spine trauma (e.g., whiplash injury, fall), I decided to wait on ordering an MRI of the cervical spine.

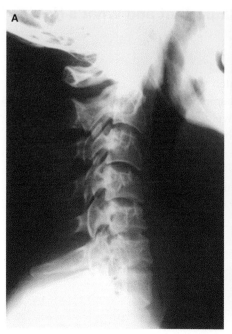
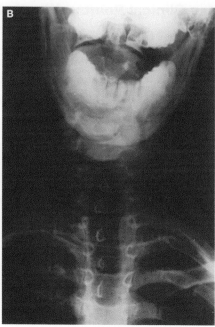

Fig. 2.2 Cervical spine radiograph. (A) Lateral cervical radiograph demonstrating straightening of the normal lordotic curve. (B) Anteroposterior cervical spine radiograph with open mouth view demonstrating no gross bony abnormality. (From Drudi FM, Spaziani et al. Diagnosis and follow-up of minor cervical trauma. *Clin Imaging* 2003;27[6]:369–376, Fig. 1.)

TEST RESULTS

Alex's cervical spine radiographs revealed mild degenerative changes and straightening of the normal cervical lordotic curve (Fig. 2.2).

 Clinical Correlation—Putting It All Together

What is the diagnosis?
- Cervical strain

The Science Behind the Diagnosis

Acute cervical strain is a constellation of symptoms consisting of nonradicular neck pain that radiates in a nondermatomal pattern into the shoulders and interscapular region; headache often accompanies these symptoms. Cervical strain is usually the result of overuse injury, trauma, and stretch injury to associated muscles and ligaments (Fig. 2.3). Cervical strain can occur from acute injuries, such as motor vehicle accident-associated whiplash injuries, or may develop over time as a result of repetitive stress or overuse injuries.

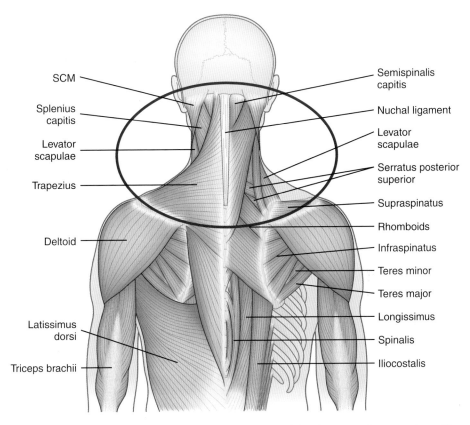

SCM

Splenius
capitis

Levator
scapulae

Trapezius

Deltoid

Latissimus
dorsi

Triceps brachii

Semispinalis
capitis

Nuchal ligament

Levator
scapulae

Serratus posterior
superior

Supraspinatus

Rhomboids

Infraspinatus

Teres minor

Teres major

Longissimus

Spinalis

Iliocostalis

Fig. 2.3   The muscles and ligaments of the neck are subject to injury from acute trauma and repetitive stress and overuse.

The trapezius is most commonly affected muscle, with resultant spasm and limited range of motion of the cervical spine (Fig. 2.4). Given that over 93% of the world's population uses smartphones, it is not surprising that there has been an increased incidence of cervical strain resulting from poor posture while looking down at the smartphone creen. The relationship of the angle of the cervical spine and the device screen can be quantified using a cumulative average of tilt angles of the neck over time. If the observed tilt angle is excessive, then significant strain is being placed on the cervical spine and soft tissues (Fig. 2.5). The pathologic lesions responsible for this clinical syndrome may emanate from the soft tissues, facet joints, or intervertebral discs.

MANAGEMENT AND TREATMENT

Cervical strain is best treated using a multimodality approach (Box 2.1). Physical therapy, including heat modalities and deep sedative massage, combined with

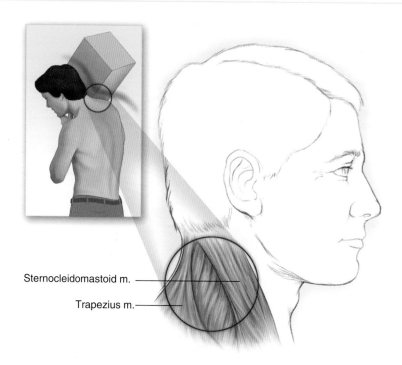

Fig. 2.4   Cervical strain is often caused by trauma to the cervical spine and adjacent soft tissues. (From Waldman SD. *Atlas of Common Pain Syndromes*. 4th ed. Philadelphia: Elsevier; 2019: Fig. 18.1.)

Sternocleidomastoid m.

Trapezius m.

simple analgesics, nonsteroidal antiinflammatory drugs, and skeletal muscle relaxants, is a reasonable starting point. Identification and correction of abnormal ergonomic factors contributing to repetitive stress and overuse injuries are key to successful treatment of cervical strain. If myofascial trigger points are identified, trigger point injections may be useful. The use of botulinum toxin A trigger point injections may offer symptomatic relief in selected patients. Gentle manipulative therapy is a useful adjunct in the management of cervical strain. The use of a soft cervical collar is discouraged because it may contribute to weakening of the cervical muscles. Opioid analgesics should be avoided in this patient population.

In patients who do not respond to conservative treatment, cervical epidural block, blockade of the medial branch of the dorsal ramus, or intraarticular injection of the facet joint with local anesthetic and steroid is extremely effective and may be a reasonable next step. Underlying sleep disturbance and depression are best treated with a tricyclic antidepressant, such as nortriptyline, which can be started at a single bedtime dose of 25 mg. The tricyclic antidepressants should be used with care in the elderly.

Correct posture   Bad posture: Cervical spine under strain

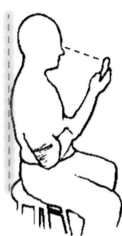 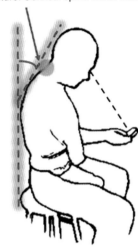

Fig. 2.5 Poor posture and an excessive tilt angle of the neck when using a smartphone may result in cervical strain. (From Lamonaca F, Polimeni G, Barbé K, et al. Health parameters monitoring by smartphone for quality of life improvement. *Measurement* 2015;73:82–94, Fig. 7.)

BOX 2.1 ■ Treatment Modalities for Cervical Strain

- Physical Modalities
  - Physical therapy
  - Local heat
  - Deep sedative massage
  - Ice rubs
- Medication Management
  - Simple analgesics
  - Nonsteroidal antiinflammatory agents
  - Skeletal muscle relaxants
- Acupuncture
- Manipulative therapy
- Interventional Pain Management
  - Trigger point injections
  - Medial branch block
  - Cervical epidural block

HIGH-YIELD TAKEAWAYS

- The patient's symptomatology is the result of repetitive stress or overuse injury rather than acute trauma, making bony abnormality unlikely.
- The patient's pain is localized in the posterior neck, shoulders, and occipital region without radiation into the upper extremities, which would be more suggestive of cervical radiculopathy.
- The patient is afebrile, making an infectious etiology unlikely.
- The patient's neurologic examination is normal; specifically, there is no sensory deficit or weakness and deep tendon reflexes are normal; making a diagnosis of cervical radiculopathy unlikely.
- There are no bowel or bladder symptoms or pathologic reflexes suggestive of myelopathy.
- The patient has significant sleep disturbance.

Suggested Readings

Han H, Shin G. Head flexion angle when web-browsing and texting using a smart-phone while walking. *Appl Ergonomics*. 2019;81:284–287.

Hudgins TH, Origenes AK, Pleuhs F, Alleva JT. Cervical sprain or strain. In: Frontera WR, Silver JK, Rizzo TD, eds. *Essentials of Physical Medicine and Rehabilitation*. 4th ed. Philadelphia: Elsevier; 2020:29–32.

Vasavada AN, Nevins DD, Monda SM, Hughes E, Lin DC. Gravitational demand on the neck musculature during tablet computer use. *Ergonomics*. 2015;58(6):990–1004.

Verwoerd M, Wittink H, Maissan F, de Raaij E, Rob JEM. Smeets. Prognostic factors for persistent pain after a first episode of nonspecific idiopathic, non-traumatic neck pain: a systematic review. *Musculoskelet Sci Pract*. 2019;42:13–37.

Waldman SD, ed. Cervical strain. In: *Atlas of Common Pain Syndromes*. 4th ed. Philadelphia: Elsevier; 2019:67–70.

Manny Perez

A 48-Year-Old Male With Neck Pain Radiating Into the Right Shoulder

- Learn the common causes of cervical radiculopathy.
- Learn the clinical presentation of cervical radiculopathy.
- Learn how to use physical examination to determine which cervical spinal nerve roots are subserving the patient's pain.
- Learn to distinguish cervical strain from cervical radiculopathy.
- Learn the important anatomic structures in cervical radiculopathy.
- Develop an understanding of the treatment options for cervical radiculopathy.
- Learn to identify red flags waving in patients who present with cervical radiculopathy.
- Develop an understanding of the role of interventional pain management in the treatment of cervical radiculopathy.

Manny Perez

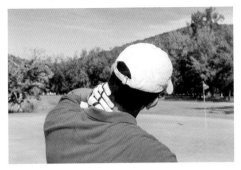

Manny Perez is a 43-year-old man with a chief complaint of, "I have neck pain with electric shocks shooting into my right shoulder." The pain began acutely five days ago after Manny was playing golf.

He denied any previous history of neck or right shoulder pain. He worked as the manager of a local Chevrolet dealership. When asked to use one finger to point to the area of the worst pain, he pointed to his neck and then his right shoulder and anterolateral arm. He then volunteered, "You know, this may sound crazy, but the top of my shoulder and upper arm kind of feels like it's gone to sleep." I told him it wasn't crazy and that we would get it figured out.

On physical examination, Manny was afebrile and normotensive. His head, ears, eyes, nose, and throat (HEENT) examination was normal, as was his cardio-pulmonary examination. His abdominal examination revealed no abnormal mass or organomegaly. There was no peripheral edema. Manny was holding his neck stiffly so as not to move it. His right shoulder was elevated in an effort to splint the neck. Palpation of the posterior neck muscles revealed tenderness to deep palpation and spasm of the paraspinous muscles, the right greater than the left. Manny cried out in pain with flexion and extension of his cervical spine. A careful neurologic examination of the upper extremities revealed a normal examination result on the left, but decreased sensation over the deltoid and anterolateral upper extremity on the right. Because of his neck spasm, it was difficult to perform a motor examination, but there was a suggestion of subtle weakness of the biceps and deltoid muscles on the right. The biceps reflex was normal on the left, but definitely diminished on the right. His brachioradialis and triceps reflexes were physiologic bilaterally. Lower extremity motor and sensory examination, as well as lower extremity deep tendon reflexes, were normal. The Spurling test was positive (see Fig. 2.1). No pathologic reflexes or clonus were identified. Manny denied bowel and bladder symptoms associated with his pain.

Key Clinical Points—What's Important and What's Not

THE HISTORY

- History of acute trauma: a golfing injury
- No history of previous neck pain

- Neck pain with pain radiating into the shoulder and upper extremity
- Sensation that shoulder and upper arm "had gone to sleep"
- No bowel or bladder symptomatology

THE PHYSICAL EXAMINATION

- The patient is afebrile
- Neck posturing in an attempt to splint neck
- Shoulder elevation on affected side to protect and splint neck
- Diminished biceps reflex on right
- Decreased sensation over the deltoid and anterolateral upper extremity on the right
- Weakness of the deltoid and biceps muscles on the right
- Normal left upper and lower extremity motor and sensory examination
- No pathologic reflexes
- No clonus
- Positive Spurling sign

OTHER FINDINGS OF NOTE

- Normal cardiovascular examination
- Normal pulmonary examination
- Normal abdominal examination
- No peripheral edema

 ## What Tests Would You Order?

The following tests were ordered:
- MRI of the cervical spine
- EMG and nerve conduction velocity testing was deferred because of the short duration of the patient's pain; also, these tests are not diagnostic until two weeks after the onset of neural compromise

TEST RESULTS

The MRI scan of Manny's cervical spine revealed a large right-sided lateral disk herniation at C5 (Fig. 3.1). As expected, the large lateral herniated disk at C4-C5 was compressing the C5 nerve root on the right. No evidence is seen of demyelinating disease or abnormality of the cervical spinal cord.

 ## Clinical Correlation—Putting It All Together

What is the diagnosis?
- C5 radiculopathy on right

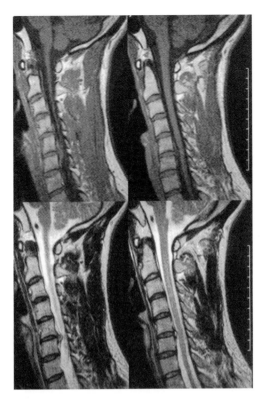

Fig. 3.1 MRI of the cervical spine demonstrating C5-C6 disc herniations. Sagittal T1-weighted *(top)* and T2-weighted *(bottom)* magnetic resonance images showing lateral C5–C6 disc extrusions. (From Kobayashi N, Asamoto S, Doi H, et al. Spontaneous regression of herniated cervical disc. *Spine J.* 2003;3(2):171–173, Fig. 1.)

The Science Behind the Diagnosis

THE DERMATOMES AND MYOTOMES

In humans, the innervation of the skin, muscles, and deep structures is determined embryologically at an early stage of fetal development, and there is amazingly little intersubject variability. Each segment of the spinal cord and its corresponding spinal nerves have a consistent segmental relationship that allows the clinician to ascertain the probable spinal level of dysfunction based on the pattern of pain, muscle weakness, and deep tendon reflex changes.

Fig. 3.2 is a dermatome chart that the clinician will find useful in determining the specific spinal level subserving a patient's pain. In general, the cervical spinal segments move down the upper extremity from cephalad to caudad on the lateral border of the upper extremity and from caudad to cephalad on the medial border.

In general, in humans, the more proximal the muscle, the more cephalad the spinal segment, with the ventral muscles innervated by higher spinal segments than the corresponding dorsal muscles. It should be remembered that pain

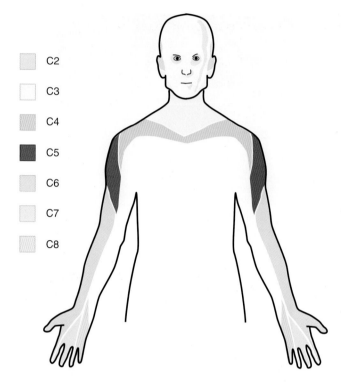

Fig. 3.2   The cervical dermatomes. (From Waldman SD. *Physical Diagnosis of Pain: An Atlas of Signs and Symptoms.* 3rd ed. St. Louis: Elsevier; 2016; Fig. 9.1.)

perceived in the region of a given muscle or joint may not be coming from the muscle or joint, but simply be referred by problems at the same cervical spinal segment that innervates the muscles.

Furthermore, the clinician needs to be aware that the relative consistent pattern of dermatomal and myotomal distribution breaks down when the pain is perceived in the deep structures of the upper extremity (e.g., the joints and tendinous insertions). With pain in these regions, the clinician should refer to a sclerotomal chart.

The concept of diagnosing a problem at a specific neurologic level via physical examination has its basis in the fact that pathology at the cervical spinal cord or cervical nerve root level manifests itself in a relatively consistent manner by dysfunction, numbness, and pain of the upper extremity, which occurs in a dermatomal distribution. Although not foolproof, a careful physical examination of the upper extremity with an eye to the neurologic level affected can frequently guide the clinician in designing a more targeted workup and treatment plan. By overlapping the information gleaned from physical examination with the neuroanatomic information gained from magnetic resonance imaging and the

TABLE 3.1 ■ Clinical Features of Cervical Radiculopathy

Cervical Root	Location of Pain	Sensory Deficit	Weakness	Reflex Changes
C5	Neck, shoulder, anterolateral arm	Numbness in deltoid area	Deltoid and biceps	Biceps reflex
C6	Neck, shoulder, lateral aspect of arm	Dorsolateral aspect of thumb and index finger	Biceps, wrist extensors, pollicis longus, index finger	Brachioradialis reflex
C7	Neck, shoulder, lateral aspect of arm, dorsal forearm	Index and middle fingers and dorsum of hand	Triceps	Triceps reflex

neurophysiologic information from electromyography, a highly accurate diagnosis can be made as to which level of the cervical spine is responsible for the patient's symptoms.

Testing for the C5 dermatome is best carried out by a careful sensory evaluation of the lateral aspect of the more cephalad portion of the upper extremity (see Fig. 3.2). Decreased sensation in this anatomic region can be ascribed to proximal lesions of the spinal cord, such as a syrinx; more distal lesions of the C5 nerve root, such as impingement by a herniated disc; or a lesion of the more peripheral axillary nerve. For this reason, correlation with manual muscle testing and evaluation of the deep tendon reflex, combined with radiographic and electromyographic testing, can help to determine the exact site of pathology (Table 3.1).

Testing for the C5 myotome is best carried out by manual muscle testing of the deltoid muscle. The deltoid muscle is primarily innervated by the C5 nerve, with a small contribution in most patients from the C6 nerve. Because in most patients abduction of the deltoid is a C5 function, the muscle should be tested as follows. The patient is placed in the standing position with the affected extremity resting against the patient's side. The patient is asked to flex the elbow to 90 degrees and then asked to abduct the affected extremity forcefully at the shoulder (Fig. 3.3). If the manual muscle testing is normal, the examiner should not be able to resist abduction nor be able to force the arm back toward the patient's side. If the patient has primary shoulder pathology that precludes this test, the clinician may test the strength of flexion of the biceps, which is also primarily innervated by C5.

The biceps deep tendon reflex is mediated via the C5 spinal segment. To test the biceps reflex, the patient is asked to relax and lay the affected extremity against the clinician's arm. The clinician then strikes the biceps tendon at the elbow with a neurologic hammer and grades the response (see Fig. 3.3). A diminished or absent reflex might point to compromise of the C5 segment, whereas a hyperactive response might suggest an upper motor neuron lesion, such as cervical myelopathy.

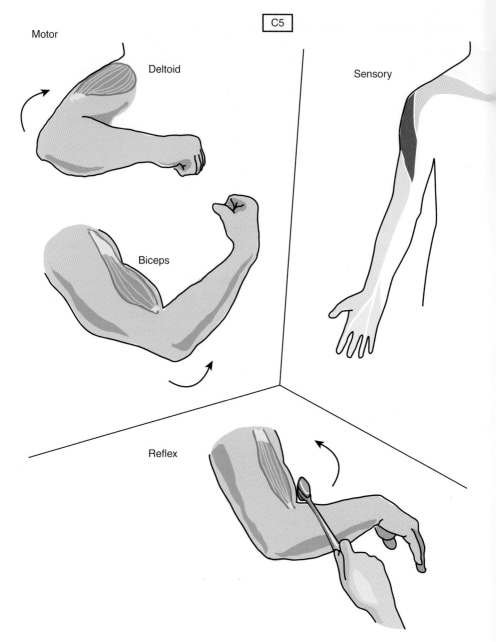

Fig. 3.3 Testing the C5 dermatome and myotome. (From Waldman S: *Physical Diagnosis of Pain: An Atlas of Signs and Symptoms*. 3rd ed. St. Louis: 2016; Elsevier, Fig. 9.2.)

CERVICAL RADICULOPATHY

Cervical radiculopathy is a constellation of symptoms consisting of neurogenic neck and upper extremity pain emanating from the cervical nerve roots. In addition to pain, the patient may experience numbness, weakness, and loss of reflexes. These symptoms are usually unilateral. The C6 and C7 nerve roots are most commonly affected. The causes of cervical radiculopathy include herniated disc, foraminal stenosis, tumor, osteophyte formation, and rarely, infection. The age-adjusted incidence of cervical radiculopathy is 83 per 100,00 persons, with smoking, axial load bearing, female gender, White race, and the arthridities being predisposing factors.

Patients suffering from cervical radiculopathy complain of pain, numbness, tingling, and paresthesias in the distribution of the affected nerve root or roots (see Table 3.1). Patients may also note weakness and lack of coordination in the affected extremity. Muscle spasms and neck pain, as well as pain referred to the trapezius and interscapular region, are common. Decreased sensation, weakness, and reflex changes are demonstrated on physical examination. Spurling test will often exacerbate the pain of cervical radiculopathy. This test is performed by asking the patient to extend and laterally rotate the cervical spine while the physician applies an axial load (see Fig. 2.1).

Cervical radiculopathy is a clinical diagnosis supported by a combination of clinical history, physical examination, radiography, and MRI. Pain syndromes that may mimic cervical radiculopathy include cervicalgia, cervical bursitis, cervical fibromyositis, inflammatory arthritis, cardiac pain, acute herpes zoster of the cervical dermatomes, entrapment syndromes of the upper extremity thoracic outlet syndrome, and disorders of the cervical spinal cord, roots, plexus, and nerves (Fig. 3.4, Table 3.2).

THE INTERVERTEBRAL DISC

The cervical intervertebral disc has two major functions. The first is to serve as the major shock-absorbing structure of the cervical spine, and the second is to facilitate the synchronized movement of the cervical spine and, at the same time, helping to prevent impingement of the neural structures and vasculature that traverse the cervical spine. Both the shock-absorbing function and the movement/protective function of the cervical intervertebral disc are functions of the disc structure as well as of the laws of physics that affect it.

To understand how the cervical intervertebral disc functions in health and becomes dysfunctional in disease, it is useful to think of the disc as a closed, fluid-filled container. The outside of the container is made up of a top and

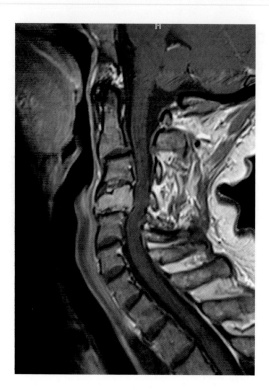

Fig. 3.4 T1-weighted magnetic resonance image showing relation of a metastatic spinal tumor to the cervical spinal cord. (From Molina CA, Gokaslan ZL, Sciubba DM. Diagnosis and management of metastatic cervical spine tumors. *Orthop Clin North Am*. 2012;43[1]:75—87.)

TABLE 3.2 ■ Clinical Syndromes That Can Mimic Cervical Radiculopathy

Clinical Condition	Signs and Symptoms
Cervical myelopathy	Decreased manual dexterity, gait changes, bowel or bladder dysfunction, upper motor neuron findings (e.g., Hoffman sign)
Acute herpes zoster	Pain preceding rash in affected cervical dermatomes
Cardiogenic pain	Radiating pain into the left shoulder and upper extremity
Parsonage-Turner syndrome	Acute onset of upper extremity pain, usually followed by weakness and sensory disturbances
Entrapment of the peripheral nerves of the upper extremities	Sensory deficits and weakness in the distribution of the affected peripheral nerve
Thoracic outlet syndrome	Pain and weakness of the lower brachial plexus secondary to nerve root compression

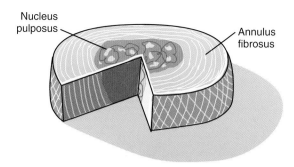

Fig. 3.5 The cervical intervertebral disc can be thought of as a closed, fluid-filled container. (From Waldman SD. *Physical Diagnosis of Pain: An Atlas of Signs and Symptoms.* 3rd ed. St. Louis: Elsevier; 2016: Fig. 2-1.)

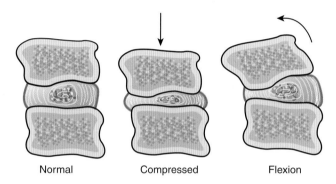

Fig. 3.6 The cervical intervertebral disc is a strong, yet flexible structure, shown here in the range of motion of the cervical spine. (From Waldman SD. *Pain Review.* Philadelphia: Saunders; 2009: Fig 21.2.)

bottom called the endplates, which are composed of relatively inflexible hyaline cartilage. The sides of the cervical intervertebral disc are made up of a woven crisscrossing matrix of fibroelastic fibers that tightly attaches to the top and bottom endplates. This woven matrix of fibers is called the annulus, and it completely surrounds the sides of the disc (Fig. 3.5). The interlaced structure of the annulus results in an enclosing mesh that is extremely strong, yet is very flexible, which facilitates the compression of the disc during the wide range of motion of the cervical spine (Fig. 3.6).

Inside of this container consisting of the top and bottom endplates and surrounding annulus is the water-containing mucopolysaccharide gel-like substance called the nucleus pulposus (see Fig. 3.5). The nucleus is incompressible and transmits any pressure placed on one portion of the disc to the surrounding nucleus. In health, the water-filled gel creates a positive intradiscal pressure,

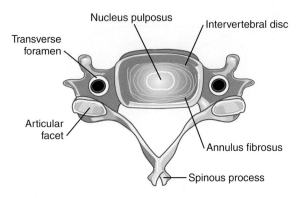

Fig. 3.7 Various types of disc degeneration and herniation. (From Waldman SD. *Pain Review*. Philadelphia: Saunders; 2009: Fig. 21.3.)

which forces apart the adjacent vertebra and helps protect the spinal cord and exiting nerve roots. When the cervical spine moves, the incompressible nature of the nucleus pulposus maintains a constant intradiscal pressure, whereas some fibers of the disc relax and others contract.

As the cervical intervertebral disc ages, it becomes less vascular and loses its ability to absorb water into the disc. This results in degradation of the disc's shock-absorbing and motion-facilitating functions. This problem is made worse by degeneration of the annulus, which allows portions of the disc wall to bulge, distorting the ability of the nucleus pulposus to distribute evenly the forces placed on it throughout the entire disc. This exacerbates disc dysfunction and can contribute to further disc deterioration, which may ultimately lead to actual complete disruption of the annulus and extrusion of the nucleus (Fig. 3.7). The deterioration of the disc is responsible for many of the painful conditions emanating from the cervical spine encountered in clinical practice.

MANAGEMENT AND TREATMENT

Cervical radiculopathy is best treated with a multimodality approach. Physical therapy, including heat modalities and deep sedative massage, combined with nonsteroidal antiinflammatory drugs and skeletal muscle relaxants, is a reasonable starting point. The addition of cervical epidural nerve blocks is a logical next step. Cervical epidural blocks with local anesthetic and steroid are extremely effective in the treatment of cervical radiculopathy (Fig. 3.8). In patients who fail to respond to epidural steroid injections, a trial of spinal cord stimulation is a reasonable next step if definitive surgical treatment is not an option. Percutaneous disc decompression and open surgical discectomy are indicated for patients who fail to respond to more conservative measures (Fig. 3.9).

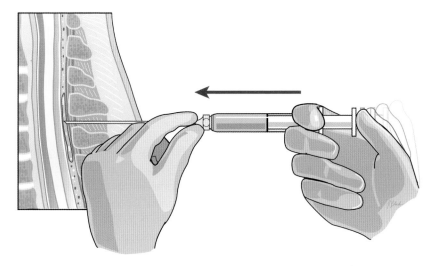

Fig. 3.8 Cervical epidural block. (From Waldman SD. *Atlas of Interventional Pain Management*. 4th ed. Philadelphia: Saunders; 2015: Fig. 44.9.)

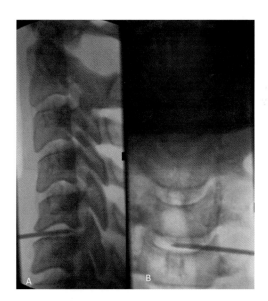

Fig. 3.9 Patient with symptomatic C5—C6 intervertebral disc herniation underwent fluoroscopic-guided percutaneous mechanical decompression (mechanical high rotation per minute device with spiral tips). (A) Lateral fluoroscopic view illustrating the decompressor located in the posterior third of the intervertebral disc. (B) A—P fluoroscopic view illustrating the decompressor placed in the midline at midway between the two vertebral endplates. (From Kelekis A, Filippiadis DK. Percutaneous treatment of cervical and lumbar herniated disc. *Eur J Radiol*. 2015; 84(5):771—776, Fig. 2.)

HIGH-YIELD TAKEAWAYS

- The patient is afebrile, making an acute infectious etiology (e.g., epidural abscess) unlikely.
- The patient's symptomatology is the result of acute trauma to the cervical intervertebral disc.
- The patient's pain is localized in the neck, right shoulder, and anterolateral upper extremity, which is highly suggestive of cervical radiculopathy.
- The patient's symptoms are unilateral, which would be more suggestive of cervical radiculopathy.
- The patient's neurologic examination is abnormal in the affected right upper extremity with a C5 sensory deficit, deltoid and biceps weakness, and a diminished biceps reflex, which is highly suggestive of a right C5 radiculopathy.
- There are no bowel or bladder symptoms or pathologic reflexes suggestive of myelopathy.
- MRI scanning is highly sensitive in the diagnosis of discogenic disease and is useful in ruling out other space-occupying lesions that may be producing radicular symptoms (see Fig. 3.4).

Suggested Readings

Corey DL, Comeau D. Cervical radiculopathy. *Med Clin North Am.* 2014;98(4):791–799.
Leveque J-CA, Marong-Ceesay B, Cooper T, Howe CR. Diagnosis and treatment of cervical radiculopathy and myelopathy. *Phys Med Rehabil Clin North Am.* 2015;26 (3):491–511.
Waldman SD. Cervical epidural nerve block: The translaminar approach. In: *Atlas of Interventional Pain Management.* 5th ed. Philadelphia: Elsevier; 2020.
Waldman SD. Cervical radiculopathy. In: *Pain Review.* 2nd ed. Philadelphia: Saunders; 2017:236–237.
Waldman SD. Functional anatomy of the cervical spine. In: *Physical Diagnosis of Pain: An Atlas of Signs and Symptoms.* 4th ed. Philadelphia: Elsevier; 2020.

Olga Fedorov

A 78-Year-Old Female With A 2½-Week History of Neck Pain Radiating Into the Left Upper Extremity

- Learn the common causes of cervical radiculopathy.
- Learn the clinical presentation of cervical radiculopathy.
- Learn how to use physical examination to determine which cervical spinal nerve root is compromised.
- Learn to distinguish cervical strain from cervical radiculopathy.
- Learn the important anatomic structures in cervical radiculopathy.
- Develop an understanding of the treatment options for cervical radiculopathy.
- Learn to identify red flags waving in patients who present with cervical radiculopathy.
- Develop an understanding of the role of interventional pain management in the treatment of cervical radiculopathy.

Olga Fedorov

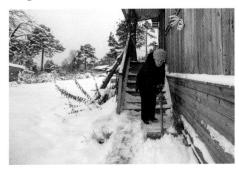

Olga Fedorov is a 78-year-old woman with a chief complaint of, "My neck and arm are killing me." Olga's pain began about 2½ weeks ago after she shoveled her back walk so her dog, Chekov, could go outside to do his business. That night, Olga found it hard to get comfortable in bed because her neck and left arm were hurting. Since that time, Olga has been sleeping sitting up in a chair. I specifically asked whether she was sleeping in a chair because she couldn't breathe or because it hurt when she tried to lie down. She glared at me and said, "Doctor . . . My breathing is just fine!" When I asked Olga to point with one finger and show me where it hurt, she pointed to her neck and the side of her left arm. She said that the pain was sharp like a knife and sometimes it would go into her thumb and index finger. She also said she was having trouble holding the cup from which she liked to drink tea. Her hand was so weak that yesterday she had dropped the pan in which she was boiling water for her tea, burning her leg.

I asked Olga what made her pain worse and she said, "Lying down and when I cough." I asked her what made the pain better and, without missing a beat, she said, "My tea with honey!" Olga denied having any problem walking to the bathroom or that she was losing any urine or feces.

On physical examination, Olga was afebrile and mildly hypertensive. Her head, ears, eyes, nose, and throat (HEENT) examination revealed dense bilateral cataracts. I asked Olga was she having any problem seeing and she said that she could see better than I could! I made a note to refer her to an ophthalmologist before she left the office. Her cardiopulmonary examination revealed a grade 2 mitral valve systolic murmur. Her abdominal examination was benign, with no abnormal mass or organomegaly. There was a trace of peripheral edema and a small healing second-degree burn on her right shin. Palpation of the posterior neck muscles revealed tenderness to deep palpation and spasm of the paraspinous muscles, left greater than right. Olga really did not want me to move her neck, but she was stoic about it. There was decreased range of motion with flexion and extension. Right lateral bending caused her to whimper. I asked what was wrong and she said that when I bent her neck that it "felt like an electric shock" in her thumb and index finger.

Findings from a careful neurologic examination of the upper extremities were normal in the right upper extremity, but sensation was decreased over the

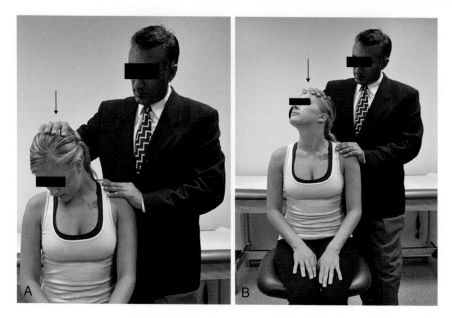

Fig. 4.1 Spurling maneuver (A) and modified Spurling maneuver (B). (From Frontera W, Silver J, Rizzo T. *Essentials of Physical Medicine and Rehabilitation*. 4th ed. Philadelphia: Elsevier; 2019: Fig. 5.3.)

dorsolateral aspect of the left thumb and index finger. Her wrist extensors on the left were surprisingly weak, as was her extensor pollicis longus muscle on the left. Her biceps deep tendon reflexes were normal bilaterally. The brachioradialis reflex was normal on the right, but only trace on the left. The triceps reflexes were also normal bilaterally. Findings from an examination of the motor, sensory, and deep tendon reflexes in both lower extremities were normal. The Spurling maneuver and modified Spurling maneuver findings were positive (Fig. 4.1). A positive Tinel's sign over the carpal tunnel was noted. Phalen's test was negative. No pathologic reflexes or clonus were identified.

Key Clinical Points—What's Important and What's Not
THE HISTORY

- History of acute trauma: onset of pain after shoveling snow
- No significant history of previous neck pain
- Neck pain with pain radiating into the upper extremity and thumb and index finger
- Complaint of inability to hold a teacup and dropping a pan of boiling water

- No bowel or bladder symptomatology
- Denies decrease in visual acuity

THE PHYSICAL EXAMINATION

- The patient is afebrile
- Spasm of paraspinous muscles, left greater than right
- Decreased range of motion of the cervical spine, with guarding
- Diminished brachioradialis reflex on left
- Decreased sensation over the dorsolateral aspect of the thumb and index finger
- Weakness of the wrist extensors, pollicis longus
- Normal right upper and bilateral lower extremity motor and sensory examination
- No pathologic reflexes
- No clonus
- Positive Spurling and modified Spurling sign
- Positive Tinel's sign over the left carpal tunnel
- Negative Phalen's test bilaterally

OTHER FINDINGS OF NOTE

- Bilateral cataracts
- Grade 2 mitral valve murmur
- Healing second-degree burn on her leg
- Mild hypertension

What Tests Would You Order?

The following tests were ordered:
- MRI scan of the cervical spine
- Electromyography and nerve conduction testing of the neck and left upper extremity

TEST RESULTS

The MRI scan of the cervical spine revealed significant degenerative changes and a large herniated disc at C6-C7 (Fig. 4.2). Electromyography of the left upper extremity revealed findings consistent with a moderate C6 radiculopathy on the left. Nerve conduction velocity testing across the left carpal tunnel revealed delayed conduction velocities, consistent with a mild carpal tunnel syndrome.

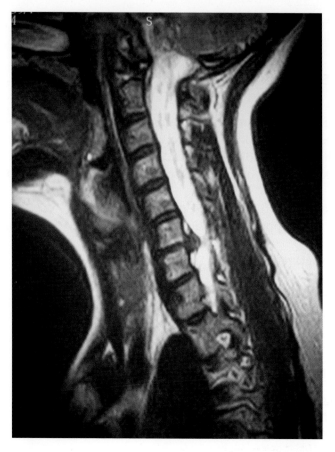

Fig. 4.2 Sagittal MRI showing C6-C7 disc degeneration and a large herniation. (From Maxey L, Magnusson J. *Rehabilitation for the Postsurgical Orthopedic Patient*. 3rd ed. St. Louis: Mosby; 2013: Fig. 14.2.)

Clinical Correlation—Putting It All Together

What is the diagnosis?
- C6 radiculopathy
- Mild carpal tunnel syndrome
- Bilateral cataracts

The Science Behind the Diagnosis

THE DERMATOMES AND MYOTOMES

In humans, the innervation of the skin, muscles, and deep structures is determined embryologically at an early stage of fetal development, with amazingly

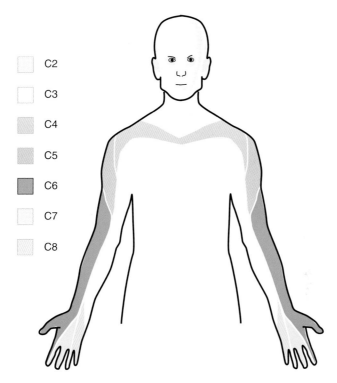

Fig. 4.3 The cervical dermatomes. (From Waldman SD. *Physical Diagnosis of Pain: An Atlas of Signs and Symptoms*. 3rd ed. St. Louis: Elsevier; 2016: Fig. 10.1.)

little intersubject variability. Each segment of the spinal cord and its corresponding spinal nerves have a consistent segmental relationship that allows the clinician to ascertain the probable spinal level of dysfunction based on the pattern of pain, muscle weakness, and deep tendon reflex changes.

Fig. 4.3 is a dermatome chart that the clinician can use to determine the specific spinal level subserving a patient's pain. In general, the cervical spinal segments move down the upper extremity from cephalad to caudad on the lateral border of the upper extremity and from caudad to cephalad on the medial border.

In general, in humans, the more proximal the muscle, the more cephalad the spinal segment, with the ventral muscles innervated by higher spinal segments than the corresponding dorsal muscles. It should be remembered that pain perceived in the region of a given muscle or joint may not be coming from that muscle or joint, but simply be referred by problems at the same cervical spinal segment that innervates the muscles. Furthermore, the clinician needs to be aware that the relatively consistent pattern of dermatomal and myotomal

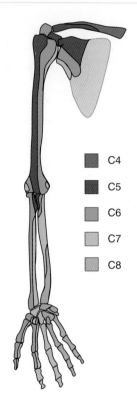

Fig. 4.4   The cervical sclerotomes. (From Waldman SD. *Physical Diagnosis of Pain: An Atlas of Signs and Symptoms*. 3rd ed. St. Louis: Elsevier; 2016: Fig. 8.2.)

distribution breaks down when the pain is perceived in the deep structures of the upper extremity (e.g., the joints and tendinous insertions). With pain in these regions, the clinician should refer to a sclerotomal chart (Fig. 4.4).

The concept of diagnosing a problem at a specific neurologic level via physical examination has its basis in the fact that pathology at the cervical spinal cord or cervical nerve root level manifests itself in a relatively consistent manner by dysfunction, numbness, and pain of the upper extremity, which occurs in a dermatomal distribution. Although not foolproof, a careful physical examination of the upper extremity, with an eye to the neurologic level affected, frequently can guide the clinician in designing a more targeted workup and treatment plan. By overlapping the information gleaned from physical examination with the neuroanatomic information gained from MRI and the neurophysiologic information from electromyography, a highly accurate diagnosis can be made as to what level of the cervical spine is responsible for the patient's symptoms.

Testing for the C6 dermatome is best carried out by a careful sensory evaluation of the lateral aspect of the more distal portion of the upper extremity (see

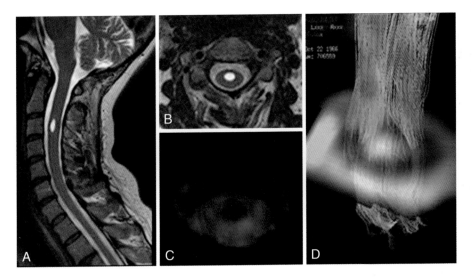

Fig. 4.5 Focal syrinx of the cervical spinal cord in a patient with cervical myelopathy. Sagittal (A) and axial (B) T2-weighted images demonstrate a focal syrinx in the central spinal cord at the C3 level. C, Axial color-coded fractional anisotropy map demonstrates no fiber tracts running through the lesion. D, Tractography shows displacement of the fiber tracts around the syrinx. Identical tractography findings are seen with spinal cord ependymomas. In contradistinction, spinal cord astrocytoma tractography would show infiltrated or attenuated fibers traversing the lesion. (From Lerner A, Mogensen MA, Kim PE, et al. Clinical applications of diffusion tensor imaging. *World Neurosurg*. 2014;82(1−2): 96−109, Fig. 3.)

Fig. 4.3). Decreased sensation in this anatomic region can be ascribed to proximal lesions of the spinal cord, such as a syrinx; more distal lesions of the C6 nerve root, such as impingement by a herniated disc; or a lesion of the more peripheral portion of the nerve (Fig. 4.5). For this reason, correlation with manual muscle testing and evaluation of the deep tendon reflex combined with radiographic and electromyographic testing can help to determine the exact site of the pathology.

Testing for the C6 myotome is best carried out by manual muscle testing of the radial wrist extensors. The radial wrist extensors are primarily innervated by the C6 nerve. Because extension on the radial aspect of the wrist is a C6 function, with C7 providing innervation for the ulnar wrist extensor, C6 integrity should be tested as follows. The patient is placed in the sitting position with the fingers slightly flexed to avoid any extensor activity of the muscles of finger extension. The patient is then asked to extend the wrist in a radial direction while the clinician applies resistance (Fig. 4.6). If the finding of the manual muscle testing for the C6 myotome is normal, the examiner should not be able to resist the radial wrist extension. If the C6 myotome is compromised and the C7 myotome is intact, then the clinician will observe ulnar wrist deviation on extension.

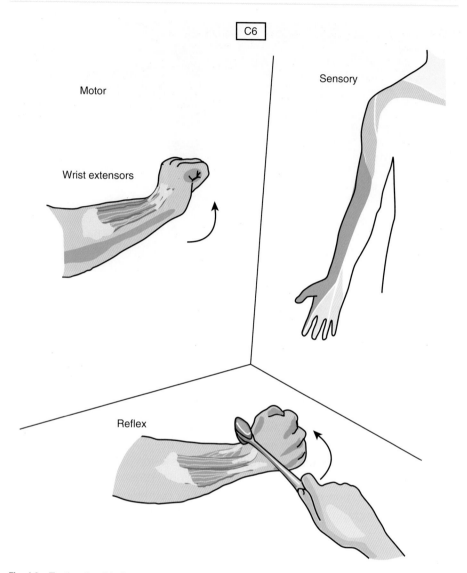

Fig. 4.6 Testing the C6 dermatome and myotome. (From Waldman SD. *Physical Diagnosis of Pain: An Atlas of Signs and Symptoms*. 3rd ed. St. Louis: Elsevier; 2016: Fig. 10.3.)

The brachioradialis deep tendon reflex is mediated via the C6 spinal segment. To test the brachioradialis reflex, the patient is asked to relax and lay the affected extremity against the clinician's arm. The clinician then strikes the brachioradialis tendon with a neurologic hammer and grades the response (see Fig. 4.6). A diminished or absent reflex might point to compromise of the C6 segment, whereas a hyperactive response might suggest an upper motor neuron lesion, such as cervical myelopathy.

TABLE 4.1 ■ **Clinical Features of Cervical Radiculopathy**

Cervical Root	Pain Location	Sensory Deficit	Weakness	Reflex Changes
C5	Neck, shoulder, anterolateral arm	Numbness in deltoid area	Deltoid and biceps	Biceps reflex
C6	Neck, shoulder, lateral aspect of arm	Dorsolateral aspect of thumb and index finger	Biceps, wrist extensors, pollicis longus, index finger	Brachioradialis reflex
C7	Neck, shoulder, lateral aspect of arm, dorsal forearm	Index and middle fingers and dorsum of hand	Triceps	Triceps reflex

CERVICAL RADICULOPATHY

Cervical radiculopathy is a constellation of symptoms consisting of neurogenic neck and upper extremity pain emanating from the cervical nerve roots. In addition to pain, the patient may experience numbness, weakness, and loss of reflexes. These symptoms are usually unilateral. The C6 and C7 nerve roots are most commonly affected. The causes of cervical radiculopathy include herniated disc, foraminal stenosis, tumor, osteophyte formation, and rarely, infection. The age-adjusted incidence of cervical radiculopathy is 83 per 100,00 persons, with smoking, axial load bearing, female gender, white race, and the arthridities being predisposing factors.

Patients suffering from cervical radiculopathy complain of pain, numbness, tingling, and paresthesias in the distribution of the affected nerve root or roots (see Table 4.1). Patients may also note weakness and lack of coordination in the affected extremity. Muscle spasms and neck pain, as well as pain referred to the trapezius and interscapular region, are common. Decreased sensation, weakness, and reflex changes are demonstrated on physical examination. The Spurling maneuver will often exacerbate the pain of cervical radiculopathy. This test is performed by asking the patient to extend and laterally rotate the cervical spine while the physician applies an axial load (see Fig. 4.1).

Cervical radiculopathy is a clinical diagnosis supported by a combination of clinical history, physical examination, radiography, and MRI. Pain syndromes that may mimic cervical radiculopathy include cervicalgia, cervical bursitis, cervical fibromyositis, inflammatory arthritis, cardiac pain, acute herpes zoster of the cervical dermatomes, and entrapment syndromes of the upper extremity including thoracic outlet syndrome, as well as disorders of the cervical spinal cord, roots, plexus, and nerves (Fig. 4.7; Table 4.2).

THE INTERVERTEBRAL DISC

The cervical intervertebral disc has two major functions. The first is to serve as the major shock-absorbing structure of the cervical spine, and the

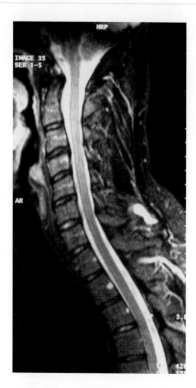

Fig. 4.7   Magnetic resonance imaging (T2) of an interspinous bursa measuring 2 × 2 × 2.5 cm between C6 and C7. (From Perka C, Schneider SV, Buttgereit F, Matziolis G. Development of cervical interspinous bursitis after prolonged sports trauma: a case report. *Joint Bone Spine.* 2006;73(1):118–120.)

TABLE 4.2 ■ Clinical Syndromes That Can Mimic Cervical Radiculopathy

Clinical Condition	Signs and Symptoms
Cervical myelopathy	Decreased manual dexterity, gait changes, bowel or bladder dysfunction, upper motor neuron findings (e.g., Hoffman sign)
Acute herpes zoster	Pain preceding rash in affected cervical dermatomes
Cardiogenic pain	Radiating pain into the left shoulder and upper extremity
Parsonage-Turner syndrome	Acute onset of upper extremity pain, usually followed by weakness and sensory disturbances
Entrapment of the peripheral nerves of the upper extremities	Sensory deficits and weakness in the distribution of the affected peripheral nerve
Thoracic outlet syndrome	Pain and weakness of the lower brachial plexus secondary to nerve root compression

second is to facilitate the synchronized movement of the cervical spine while helping to prevent impingement of the neural structures and vasculature that traverse the cervical spine. Both the shock-absorbing function and the movement/protective function of the cervical intervertebral disc are functions of the disc structure as well as of the laws of physics that affect it.

To understand how the cervical intervertebral disc functions in health and becomes dysfunctional in disease, it is useful to think of the disc as a closed fluid-filled container. The outside of the container is made up of a top and bottom called the endplates, which are composed of relatively inflexible hyaline cartilage. The sides of the cervical intervertebral disc are made up of a woven criss-crossing matrix of fibroelastic fibers that tightly attaches to the top and bottom endplates. This woven matrix of fibers is called the annulus, and it completely surrounds the sides of the disc (Fig. 4.8). The interlaced structure of the annulus results in an enclosing mesh that is extremely strong yet at the same time, very flexible, which facilitates the compression of the disc during the wide range of motion of the cervical spine (Fig. 4.9).

Inside of this container consisting of the top and bottom endplates and surrounding annulus is the water-containing mucopolysaccharide gel-like substance called the nucleus pulposus (see Fig. 4.8). The nucleus is incompressible

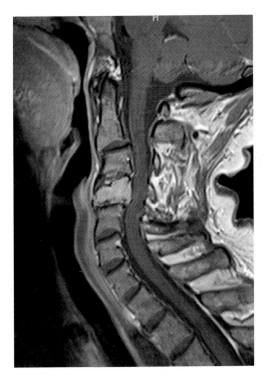

Fig. 4.8 The sides of the cervical intervertebral disc are made up of a woven crisscrossing matrix of fibroelastic fibers that tightly attaches to the top and bottom endplates. This woven matrix of fibers is called the annulus, and it completely surrounds the sides of the disc. (From Waldman SD. *Atlas of Interventional Pain Management*. 4th ed. Philadelphia: Saunders; 2015: Fig 44-2.)

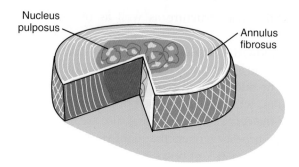

Fig. 4.9 The cervical intervertebral disc can be thought of as a closed, fluid-filled container. (From Waldman SD. *Physical Diagnosis of Pain: An Atlas of Signs and Symptoms*. 3rd ed. St. Louis: Elsevier; 2016: Fig. 2-1.)

and transmits any pressure placed on one portion of the disc to the surrounding nucleus. In health, the water-filled gel creates a positive intradiscal pressure, which forces apart the adjacent vertebra and helps protect the spinal cord and exiting nerve roots. When the cervical spine moves, the incompressible nature of the nucleus pulposus maintains a constant intradiscal pressure while some fibers of the disc relax and others contract.

As the cervical intervertebral disc ages, it becomes less vascular and loses its ability to absorb water into the disc. This results in degradation of the disc's shock-absorbing and motion-facilitating functions. This problem is made worse by degeneration of the annulus, which allows portions of the disc wall to bulge, distorting the ability of the nucleus pulposus to distribute evenly the forces placed on it throughout the entire disc. This exacerbates disc dysfunction and can contribute to further disc deterioration, which may ultimately lead to actual complete disruption of the annulus and extrusion of the nucleus (Fig. 4.10). The deterioration of the disc is responsible for many of the painful conditions emanating from the cervical spine that are encountered in clinical practice.

MANAGEMENT AND TREATMENT

Cervical radiculopathy is best treated with a multimodality approach. Physical therapy, including heat modalities and deep sedative massage, combined with nonsteroidal anti inflammatory drugs and skeletal muscle relaxants, is a reasonable starting point. The addition of cervical epidural nerve blocks is a logical next step. Cervical epidural blocks with local anesthetic and steroid are extremely effective in the treatment of cervical radiculopathy (see Fig. 3.8). In patients who fail to respond to epidural steroid injections, a trial of spinal cord stimulation is a reasonable next step if definitive surgical treatment is not an option. Percutaneous disc decompression and open surgical discectomy, with or

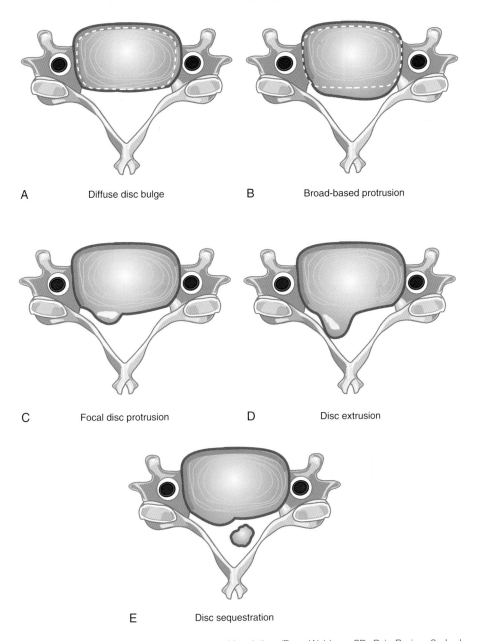

A   Diffuse disc bulge   B   Broad-based protrusion

C   Focal disc protrusion   D   Disc extrusion

E   Disc sequestration

Fig. 4.10 Various types of disc degeneration and herniation. (From Waldman SD. *Pain Review*. 2nd ed. Philadelphia: Saunders; 2017:52, Fig. 21.3.)

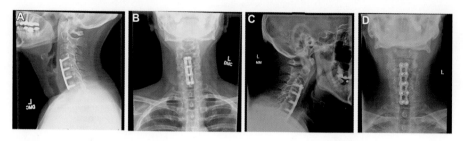

Fig. 4.11 Percutaneous disc decompression and open surgical discectomy with or without cervical fusion. (From Kim S, Alan N, Sansosti A, Agarwal N, Wecht DA. Complications after 3- and 4-level anterior cervical diskectomy and fusion. *World Neurosurg.* 2019;130:e1105–e1110, Fig. 1.)

without cervical fusion, are indicated for patients who fail to respond to more conservative measures (Fig. 4.11).

Physical findings of cervical myelopathy secondary to a herniated disc and spondylitic disease are strong indications for surgical intervention (e.g., decompressive laminectomy, anterior cervical fusion, and discectomy). Relative indications for surgical intervention include progressive neurologic deficit, recurrent radiculopathy, persistent radiculopathy, and/or severe axial neck pain that has failed to respond to aggressive conservative therapy. The more acute and severe the myelopathy, the more urgent the need for decompression of the cervical spinal cord. High-dose intravenous steroids may reduce spinal cord swelling and may also decrease the extent of permanent neurologic deficit. The clinician must always be cognizant of the fact that more than one pathologic process may be responsible for the patient's symptomatology.

HIGH-YIELD TAKEAWAYS

- The patient is afebrile, making an acute infectious etiology (e.g., epidural abscess) unlikely.
- The patient's symptomatology is the result of acute trauma to the cervical intervertebral disc.
- The patient's pain is localized in the neck, right shoulder, and anterolateral upper extremity, which is highly suggestive of cervical radiculopathy.
- The patient's symptoms are unilateral, which would be more suggestive of cervical radiculopathy.
- The patient's neurologic examination is abnormal in the affected left upper extremity with C6 sensory deficit, weakness of the wrist extensors, and a

(Continued)

diminished brachioradialis reflex, which is highly suggestive of a left C6 radiculopathy.

- There are no bowel or bladder symptoms or pathologic reflexes suggestive of myelopathy.
- MRI scanning is highly sensitive in the diagnosis of discogenic disease and is useful in ruling out other space-occupying lesions that may be producing radicular symptoms.
- Given the patient's age, co-existent degenerative disc disease and spondolytic changes may be contributing the patient's pain symptomatology.
- It is not uncommon for patients with cervical radiculopathy also to suffer from co-existent entrapment neuropathies, such as carpal tunnel syndrome. This is known as the double crush syndrome.

Suggested Readings

Corey DL, Comeau D. Cervical radiculopathy. *Med Clin North Am*. 2014;98(4):791–799.

Leveque J-C A, Marong-Ceesay B, Cooper T, Howe CR. Diagnosis and treatment of cervical radiculopathy and myelopathy. *Phys Med Rehab Clin North Am*. 2015; 26(3):491–511.

Singh S, Kumar D, Kumar S. Risk factors in cervical spondylosis. *J Clin Orthop Trauma*. 2014;5(4):221–222.

Waldman SD. Cervical epidural nerve block: the translaminar approach. In: *Atlas of Interventional Pain Management*. 5th ed. Philadelphia: Elsevier; 2020.

Waldman SD. Cervical radiculopathy. In: *Pain Review*. 2nd ed. Philadelphia: Saunders; 2017:236–237.

Waldman SD. Functional anatomy of the cervical spine. In: *Physical Diagnosis of Pain: An Atlas of Signs and Symptoms*. 4th ed. Philadelphia: Elsevier; 2020.

CHAPTER

5

Bill Miller

A 55-Year-Old Male With a 6-Week History of Neck and Left Upper Extremity Pain

LEARNING OBJECTIVES

- Learn the common causes of cervical radiculopathy.
- Learn the clinical presentation of cervical radiculopathy.
- Learn how to use physical examination to determine which cervical spinal nerve roots are involved.
- Learn to distinguish cervical strain from cervical radiculopathy.
- Learn the important anatomic structures in cervical radiculopathy.
- Develop an understanding of the treatment options for cervical radiculopathy.
- Learn to identify red flags in patients who present with cervical radiculopathy.
- Develop an understanding of the role of interventional pain management in the treatment of cervical radiculopathy.

Bill Miller

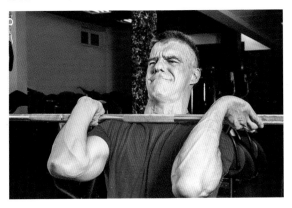

Bill Miller is a 55-year-old retired Navy SEAL with a chief complaint of, "My neck and shoulder are killing me." Bill noted that the neck pain came on acutely approximately 6 weeks ago while he was lifting weights. Gradually, despite decreased activity and simple analgesics, the pain worsened and began radiating into his shoulder and left arm. Bill had a significant past medical history of intermittent low back pain, but this was his first episode of neck pain.

While we were talking, he rested his left arm on top of his head. I had seen that posture before and it gave me a pretty good clue of what was causing Billi's pain. Ultimately, based on the clue, my guess as to what was causing Bill's pain was partially correct, but as I would soon find out, there was a lot more going on with Bill than appeared at first glance . . . so much for hoofbeats and horses! This one turned out to be a real zebra.

I asked Bill to describe what the pain felt like . . . was it sharp, dull, electric shock like, deep, aching, and he said "All of the above!" "Doc, this pain is worse than the time I got tagged with that piece of shrapnel from an IED in Afghanistan." I had heard this story several times before, but waited patiently while Bill told it one more time. "Doc, my sleep is really jacked up . . . my wife finally moved into a separate bedroom because I keep tossing and turning. Doc, you gotta help me!" I reassured him that we would get on top of his pain, but the first step was to figure out exactly what was causing it.

I asked him "What makes the pain worse?" and Bill said "Just about everything . . . any time I move my neck, take a poop, cough, try to close the door of my car . . . the pain shoots down my arm." I asked, "What makes the pain better, and he grinned and said. "Two things" . . . a bottle of Jack and putting my arm on the top of my head . . . and you know that I really hate going out and letting people see me because I know that I look like a complete idiot walking around with my hand on my head."

Bill denied any problems with urinating or defecating, difficulty walking, numbness, weakness, fever, chills . . . anything like that. Bill thought for a moment and said, "Doc, come to think of it, my balance seems off, especially when I get up to pee at night. I had been leaving the light off so I didn't wake up Meg and when I walk to the bathroom, it feels like any minute that I am going to fall. Also, I keep dropping things … Doc, lately, my walking just doesn't seem right. I can pee and poop OK, like I said, but the neck pain gets a lot worse when I take a poop. You know, I took some of my wife's pain pills from when she had a tooth pulled and those damn things constipated the hell out of me, which makes me dread trying to go to the bathroom because when I poop, it really hurts my neck and arm."

On physical examination, Bill was afebrile and normotensive. His HEENT examination was normal, as was his cardiopulmonary examination. His abdominal examination revealed no abnormal mass or organomegaly. There was no peripheral edema. I noted that Bill kept resting his left arm on top of his head (Fig. 5.1). His left shoulder was elevated in an effort to splint the neck. Palpation of the posterior neck muscles revealed tenderness to deep palpation and spasm of the paraspinous muscles, the left greater than the right. Bill really resisted my efforts to flex and extend his neck. He said, "Doc, it just hurts too damn much to move it." When I did flex his cervical spine, he cried out in pain. I asked what he felt and he said that electric shocks went down his arms. The Spurling test was positive, as was the cervical distraction test (see Fig. 2.1, Fig. 5.2). Examination of his back was unremarkable, other than a well-healed scar on the right flank from an old shrapnel wound.

A careful neurologic examination of the upper extremities was normal on the right, but there was decreased sensation over the dorsum of the hand and the index and middle fingers on the left. Because of his neck spasm, it was difficult to perform a motor examination, but Bill definitely had weakness of the triceps on the left. The biceps, brachioradialis, and triceps reflexes were normal on the right, but the left biceps reflex seemed brisk. When I tested the left brachioradialis reflex, instead of seeing the normal reflex response of elbow flexion, wrist extension, and radial wrist deviation, I observed finger flexion, which was suggestive of an inverted supinator sign. The left triceps reflex was just trace. Hoffman's sign was present on the left (Fig. 5.3). The lower extremity motor examination was normal, as was the sensory examination, but the quadriceps and Achilles reflexes were hyperactive and clonus was present bilaterally. Babinski sign was present on the left and equivocal on the right (Fig. 5.4).

I got Bill up to walk and his gait seemed a little unsteady. I performed a rectal examination and Bill's anal sphincter tone was normal. I had Bill get dressed and asked if he would like his wife to come in. He said yes, so my nurse brought Bill's wife, Meg, into the room. I told them what I thought was going on and what our next steps needed to be.

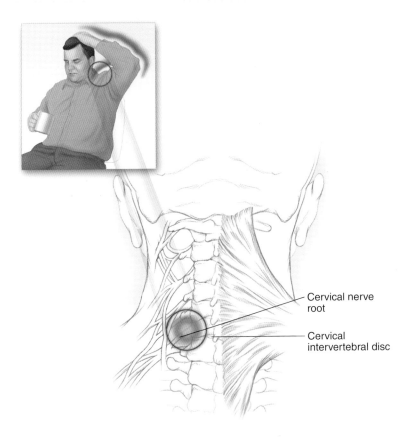

Fig. 5.1 Patients with C7 radiculopathy often place the hand of the affected extremity on the head to obtain relief. (From Waldman S. *Atlas of Common Pain Syndromes*. 4th ed. Philadelphia: Saunders; 2019; Fig. 16.1.)

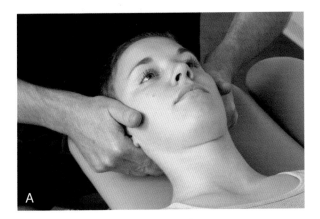

Fig. 5.2 The cervical distraction test. (From Olson K. *Manual Physical Therapy of the Spine*. 2nd ed. St. Louis: Elsevier; 2016; Fig. 6.23A.)

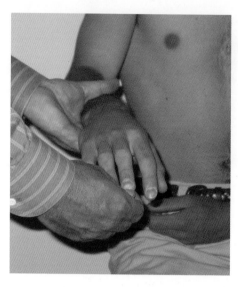

Fig. 5.3 The Hoffman test for cervical myelopathy. (From Waldman S. *Physical Diagnosis of Pain: An Atlas of Signs and Symptoms*. 3rd ed. St. Louis: Elsevier; 2016; Fig 15.1.)

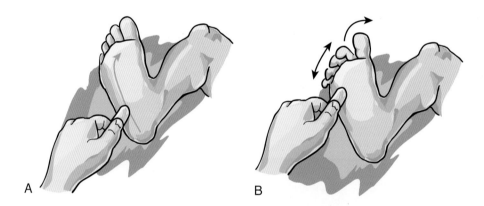

A   B

Fig. 5.4 The Babinski sign. (From Waldman S. *Physical Diagnosis of Pain: An Atlas of Signs and Symptoms*. 3rd ed. St. Louis: Elsevier; 2016; Fig. 157.1.)

Key Clinical Points—What's Important and What's Not

THE HISTORY

- History of acute trauma—injured his neck while lifting weights
- Pain and symptoms are unilateral
- Progression of pain severity

- No significant history of previous neck pain, but a history of repeated episodes of acute back pain
- Neck pain with pain radiating into the upper extremity
- Numbness of the upper extremity, dorsum of hand, and the index and middle fingers
- Complains of dropping things, gait disturbance
- Feeling unsteady, especially when walking in the dark
- Significant sleep disturbance and abnormal balance
- No bowel or bladder symptomatology, but pain on the Valsalva maneuver

THE PHYSICAL EXAMINATION

- The patient is afebrile
- Spasm of paraspinous muscles on the left greater than on the right
- Decreased range of motion of the cervical spine with guarding
- Diminished triceps reflex on left
- Decreased sensation over the dorsum of the hand and the index and middle finger on the left
- Weakness of the left triceps muscle
- Normal lower extremity motor and sensory examination
- Pathologic reflexes present including Hoffman's and Babinski signs, inverted supinator sign, hyperreflexia, and clonus
- Positive Lhermitte's sign (Fig. 5.5)
- Positive Spurling sign and cervical distraction test
- Normal anal sphincter tone

OTHER FINDINGS OF NOTE

- Well-healed scar, right flank

What Tests Would You Order?

The following tests were ordered:
- Cervical spine radiographs
- MRI of the cervicothoracic spine
- MRI of the lumbar spine
- Electromyography and nerve conduction velocity testing of the left upper extremity
- Somatosensory evoked potential testing

I also told Bill and Meg that I was going to set up an urgent consultation with a neurosurgeon because I thought Bill was probably going to need cervical spine surgery.

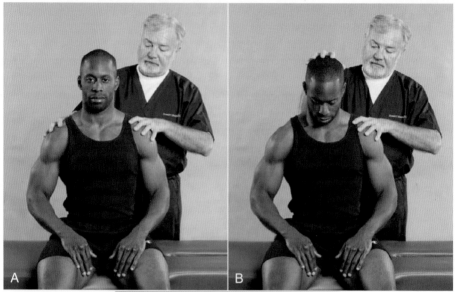

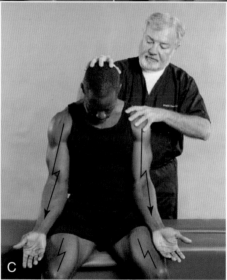

Fig. 5.5 The Lhermitte's sign. (A) The patient sits comfortably, but erect, with the head and neck in the neutral position. (B) The head and neck are passively flexed toward the chest. (C) The patient may experience a sharp, radiating pain or paresthesia along the spine and into one or more extremities. The presence of these symptoms suggests spinal cord compression or myelopathy. (From Gatterman M. *Whiplash*. St. Louis: Mosby; 2012: Fig. 4.1a-c.)

TEST RESULTS

When I received Bill's test results, I found I was right about the diagnosis, but somewhat wrong about what was causing some of Bill's symptoms. This was not a run-of-the-mill case and the MRI showed that Bill had something I had only read

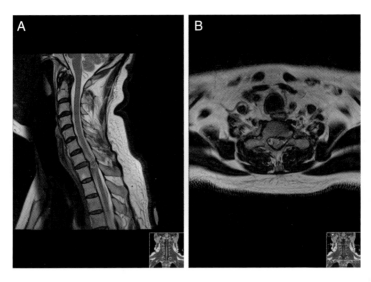

Fig. 5.6 (A) T2-weighted sagittal magnetic resonance image (MRI) of the large compressive mass at the C7—T1 junction. (B) T2-weighted axial MRI of a large compressive mass at the C7—T1 junction. (From Gunasekaran A, de los Reyes NKM, Walters J, Kazemi N: Clinical presentation, diagnosis, and surgical treatment of spontaneous cervical intradural disc herniations: a review of the literature. *World Neurosurgery* 109:275–284, 2018, Fig. 1.)

about … definitely a zebra! The MRI of the cervicothoracic spine revealed a huge C7-T1 disc extrusion on the left that tracked inferiorly. The disc extrusion was severely displacing the spinal cord both posteriorly and laterally (Fig. 5.6). But the really strange part was that on the T2-weighted axial images, the disc extrusion appeared to have extended intradurally. This certainly explained some of Bill's more worrisome symptoms and physical findings (see Fig. 5.6). The electromyography showed findings consistent with an acute C7 radiculopathy. Nerve conduction testing finding was unremarkable. Somatosensory-evoked potentials were consistent with a cervical myelopathy. Cervical spine radiographs demonstrated degenerative changes as well as disc space narrowing at C7-T1, all of which I felt were consistent with Bill's age and physically active lifestyle.

Bill's myelopathy was significant and the neurosurgeon to whom I sent Bill recommended immediate decompressive laminectomy. A wide decompressive laminectomy at C7-T1 was performed and a large cervical disc fragment was found to have migrated intradurally, causing severe compression and displacement of the cervical spinal cord (Fig. 5.7). It took the surgeon over four hours to remove the disc fragment from around the spinal cord. Once the disc fragment was removed, a large ventral dural defect through which the intervertebral disc had herniated was identified and had to be repaired (Fig. 5.8). Removal of the extruded disc decompressed the spinal cord and allowed the cord to return to a more natural alignment (Fig. 5.9). Postoperatively Bill's radiculopathic symptoms were gone and over the ensuing three months, his myelopathy resolved with physical therapy.

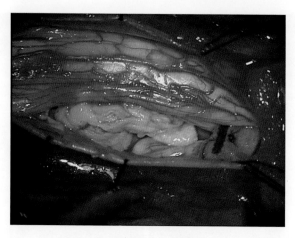

Fig. 5.7 Large intradural mass resulting in significant ventrolateral compression of the spinal cord. (From Gunasekaran A, de los Reyes NKM, Walters J, Kazemi N. Clinical presentation, diagnosis, and surgical treatment of spontaneous cervical intradural disc herniations: a review of the literature. *World Neurosurg.* 2018;109:275−284, Fig. 3.)

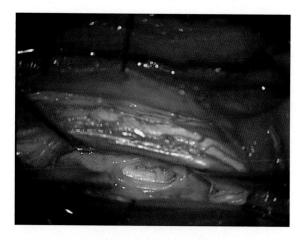

Fig. 5.8 Ventral dural defect revealing origin of intradural disc herniation. (From Gunasekaran A, de los Reyes NKM, Walters J, Kazemi N. Clinical presentation, diagnosis, and surgical treatment of spontaneous cervical intradural disc herniations: a review of the literature. *World Neurosurg.* 2018;109:275−284, Fig. 4.)

 Clinical Correlation—Putting It All Together

What is the diagnosis?
- C7 radiculopathy
- Cervical myelopathy

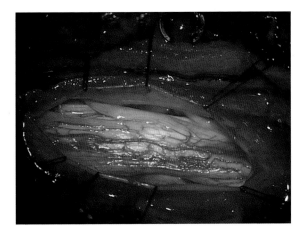

Fig. 5.9 Return of normal alignment of spinal cord after removal of large intradural disc herniation. (From Gunasekaran A, de los Reyes NKM, Walters J, et al. Clinical presentation, diagnosis, and surgical treatment of spontaneous cervical intradural disc herniations: a review of the literature. *World Neurosurg.* 2018;109:275–284, Fig. 5.)

The Science Behind the Diagnosis

CERVICAL MYELOPATHY

Cervical radiculopathy and myelopathy can exist independently or can coexist. In some patients, the signs and symptoms of cervical radiculopathy are obvious, but the signs and symptoms of myelopathy are extremely subtle. The converse can also be true. Because of the devastating impact that cervical myelopathy can have on the patient, it must be a diagnostic consideration in any patient who presents with neck pain, radiculopathy, or any symptoms suggestive of spinal cord compromise.

Cervical spondylotic myelopathy is a common degenerative condition of the cervical spine and is the most common cause of nontraumatic myelopathy in older adults (Fig. 5.10). In most instances, cervical spondylitic myelopathy is the end result of degenerative disc disease. As the cervical intervertebral discs age, mechanical stresses are placed on the cervical spine. These stresses produce osteophytes, which can impinge on nerve roots and compress the spinal cord. Associated facet arthropathy and hypertrophy of the ligamentum flavum can further contribute to the evolution of cervical spondylotic myelopathy.

Cervical myelopathy usually develops insidiously unless there is acute trauma to the cervical spine and its contents. Early symptoms may include neck pain and stiffness. Radicular pain and shock like paresthesias into the upper extremities may also develop. Often, multiple spinal segments are affected. Patients suffering from a high compressive myelopathy (C3-C5) often complain

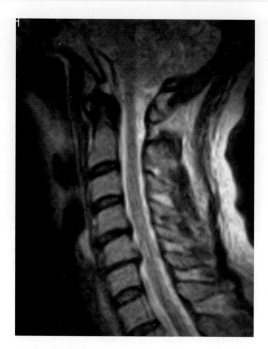

Fig. 5.10 Cervical spondolytic disease. Sagittal T2-weighted image of the cervical spine showing spinal cord compression at the C3-C4 and C4-C5 levels. At the C3-C4 level, the cord is compressed from the front and from the back. No cerebrospinal fluid is visible in the compressed regions. (From Frontera W, Silver J, Rizzo T. *Essentials of Physical Medicine and Rehabilitation*. 4th ed. Philadelphia: Elsevier; 2016: Fig. 3.2.)

of neck pain and stiffness with associated hand clumsiness and numbness. When this occurs, patients often describe difficulty in writing, dropping things, a loss of manual dexterity (e.g., inability to button a shirt or fasten a bra), and a sense that their hands "are not working right." Patients with a lower cervical myelopathy typically present with weakness, stiffness of the hands, as well as difficulty in walking, especially in the dark, owing to the loss of proprioception in the lower extremities. These patients often exhibit signs of spasticity and hyperreflexia as well as pathologic reflexes (e.g., Babinski sign, clonus, on physical examination). Urinary and bowel incontinence are less common, but difficulty fully emptying the bladder with associated frequency and hesitancy is often seen.

In patients with preexisting cervical spondylosis, acute trauma to the cervical spine, most commonly acute hyperextension injuries from motor vehicle accidents, can result in an acute cervical myelopathy. In this setting, there is often greater upper extremity weakness than lower extremity weakness, varying degrees of sensory disturbances below the lesion, and the rapid evolution of myelopathic findings, such as spasticity and urinary retention.

The concept of diagnosing a problem at a specific neurologic level via physical examination has its basis in the fact that pathology at the cervical spinal cord or cervical nerve root level manifests itself in a relatively consistent manner by dysfunction, numbness, and upper extremity pain, which occurs in a dermatomal distribution. Although not foolproof, a careful physical examination of the upper extremity with an eye to the neurologic level affected can frequently guide the clinician in designing a more targeted workup and treatment plan. By overlapping the information gleaned from physical examination with the neuroanatomic information gained from MRI and the neurophysiologic information from electromyography, a highly accurate diagnosis can be made as to what level of the cervical spine is responsible for the patient's symptoms.

CERVICAL RADICULOPATHY

Cervical radiculopathy is a constellation of symptoms consisting of neurogenic neck and upper extremity pain emanating from the cervical nerve roots. In addition to pain, the patient may experience numbness, weakness, and loss of reflexes. These symptoms are usually unilateral. The C6 and C7 nerve roots are most commonly affected. The causes of cervical radiculopathy include herniated disc, foraminal stenosis, tumor, osteophyte formation, and rarely, infection. The age-adjusted incidence of cervical radiculopathy is 83 per 100,00 persons, with smoking, axial load bearing, female gender, white race, and the arthritides being predisposing factors.

Patients suffering from cervical radiculopathy complain of pain, numbness, tingling, and paresthesias in the distribution of the affected nerve root or roots (Table 5.1). Patients may also note weakness and lack of coordination in the affected extremity. Muscle spasms and neck pain, as well as pain referred to the trapezius and interscapular region, are common. Decreased sensation, weakness, and reflex changes are demonstrated on physical examination. The Spurling test will often exacerbate the pain of cervical radiculopathy. This test is

TABLE 5.1 ■ Clinical Features of Cervical Radiculopathy

Cervical Root	Location of Pain	Sensory Deficit	Weakness	Reflex Changes
C5	Neck, shoulder, anterolateral arm	Numbness in deltoid area	Deltoid and biceps	Biceps reflex
C6	Neck, shoulder, lateral aspect of arm	Dorsolateral aspect of thumb and index finger	Biceps, wrist extensors, pollicis longus, index finger	Brachioradialis reflex
C7	Neck, shoulder, lateral aspect of arm, dorsal forearm	Index and middle fingers and dorsum of hand	Triceps	Triceps reflex

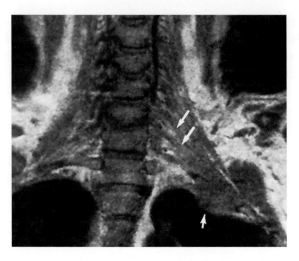

Fig. 5.11 Pancoast's tumor (adenocarcinoma) with infiltration of the brachial plexus. A 65-year-old man complained of severe pain in the shoulder radiating to the elbow, the medial side of the forearm, and the fourth and fifth fingers in an ulnar nerve distribution. Screening coronal T1-weighted MRI shows the brachial plexus from the region of the roots (*long arrows*) to the region of the trunks and divisions, where tumor invasion (*short arrow*) and loss of fat planes on the left are seen. (From Waldman SD. *Atlas of Common Pain Syndromes*. 4th ed. Philadelphia: Elsevier; 2019: Fig. 23.4.)

BOX 5.1 ■ Pain Syndromes That May Mimic Cervical Radiculopathy

- Cervicalgia
- Cervical bursitis
- Cervical fibromyositis
- Inflammatory arthritis
- Cardiac pain
- Acute herpes zoster of the cervical dermatomes
- Entrapment syndromes of the upper extremity
- Thoracic outlet syndrome
- Disorders of the cervical spinal cord, roots, plexus, and nerves

---

performed by asking the patient to extend and laterally rotate the cervical spine while the physician applies an axial load (see Fig. 4.1).

Cervical radiculopathy is a clinical diagnosis supported by a combination of clinical history, physical examination, radiography, and MRI. Pain syndromes that may mimic cervical radiculopathy include cervicalgia, cervical bursitis, cervical fibromyositis, inflammatory arthritis, cardiac pain, acute herpes zoster of the cervical dermatomes, entrapment syndromes of the upper extremity, thoracic outlet syndrome, and disorders of the cervical spinal cord, roots, plexus, and nerves (Fig. 5.11 and Box 5.1).

Testing for the C7 dermtome is best carried out by a careful sensory evaluation of the dorsum of the hand and the index and middle fingers on the affected

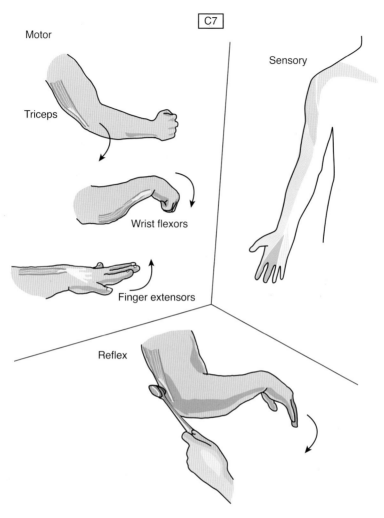

Fig. 5.12 C7 physical examination. (From Waldman SD. *Physical Diagnosis of Pain: An Atlas of Signs and Symptoms*. 3rd ed. St. Louis: Elsevier; 2016: Fig. 11.3.)

side (Fig. 5.12). Decreased sensation in this anatomic region can be ascribed to proximal lesions of the spinal cord, such as a syrinx; more distal lesions of the C7 nerve root, such as impingement by a herniated disc; or a lesion of the more peripheral portion of the nerve (Fig. 5.13). For this reason, correlation with manual muscle testing and evaluation of the deep tendon reflex combined with radiographic and electromyographic testing can help to determine the exact site of the pathology.

Testing for the C7 myotome is best carried out by manual muscle testing of the triceps muscle and the flexor carpi radialis. The wrist extensors are primarily innervated by the C7 nerve, with the flexor carpi ulnaris usually innervated by

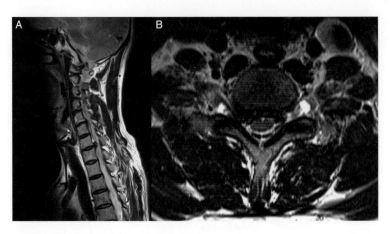

Fig. 5.13 MRI of C7-T1 herniated intervertebral disc. (A) Sagittal magnetic resonance imaging (MRI) of right foraminal disc herniation at C7—T1. (B) Axial MRI of right foraminal disc herniation at C7—T1. (From Ryu D-S, Paik H-K, Ahn S-S, et al. Herniated discs at the cervicothoracic junction. *World Neurosurg.* 2018;118:e651—e658, Fig. 3.)

C8. C7 myotome integrity should be tested as follows. The patient is placed in the sitting position with the fingers in extension to eliminate any finger flexor activity of the muscles of finger flexion. The patient is then asked to flex the wrist in a radial direction while the clinician applies resistance (see Fig. 5.12). If the manual muscle testing for the C7 myotome is normal, the examiner should not be able to resist the radial wrist flexion. If the C7 myotome is compromised and the C8 myotome is intact, then the clinician will observe ulnar wrist deviation on flexion.

The triceps deep tendon reflex is mediated via the C7 spinal segment. To test the triceps reflex, the patient is asked to relax and lay the affected extremity against the clinician's arm. The clinician then strikes the distal triceps tendon with a neurologic hammer and grades the response (see Fig. 5.12). A diminished or absent reflex might point to compromise of the C7 segment, whereas a hyperactive response might suggest an upper motor neuron lesion, such as cervical myelopathy.

MANAGEMENT AND TREATMENT

Cervical radiculopathy is best treated with a multimodality approach. Physical therapy, including heat modalities and deep sedative massage, combined with nonsteroidal anti inflammatory drugs and skeletal muscle relaxants, is a reasonable starting point. The addition of cervical epidural nerve blocks is a logical next step. Cervical epidural blocks with local anesthetic and steroid are extremely effective in the treatment of cervical radiculopathy (see Fig. 3.8). For

---

BOX 5.2 ■ Indications for Surgical Treatment of Cervical Radiculopathy and Myelopathy

- Progressive neurologic deficit
- Myelopathy
- Recurrent radiculopathy that fails to respond to aggressive conservative treatment
- Persistent radiculopathy that fails to respond to aggressive conservative treatment
- Severe axial neck pain that fails to respond to aggressive conservative therapy

---

patients who fail to respond to epidural steroid injections, a trial of spinal cord stimulation is a reasonable next step if definitive surgical treatment is not an option. Percutaneous disc decompression and open surgical discectomy, with or without cervical fusion, are indicated for patients who fail to respond to more conservative measures (see Fig. 4.11).

Physical findings of cervical myelopathy secondary to herniated disc and spondylitic disease are strong indications for surgical intervention (e.g., decompressive laminectomy, anterior cervical fusion, and discectomy). Relative indications for surgical intervention include progressive neurologic deficit, recurrent radiculopathy, persistent radiculopathy, and/or severe axial neck pain that has failed to respond to aggressive conservative therapy. The more acute and severe the myelopathy, the more urgent the need for decompression of the cervical spinal cord. High-dose intravenous steroids may reduce spinal cord swelling and may decrease the extent of permanent neurologic deficit. The clinician must always be cognizant of the fact that more than one pathologic process may be responsible for the patient's symptomatology (Box 5.2).

HIGH-YIELD TAKEAWAYS

- The patient is afebrile, making an acute infectious etiology (e.g., epidural abscess) unlikely.
- The patient's symptomatology is the result of acute trauma to the cervical intervertebral disc.
- The patient's pain is localized in the neck, right shoulder, and upper extremity, which is highly suggestive of cervical radiculopathy.
- The patient's symptoms are unilateral, which would be more suggestive of cervical radiculopathy.
- The patient's neurologic examination is abnormal in the affected left upper extremity with a C7 sensory deficit, weakness of the wrist flexors and triceps, and a diminished left triceps reflex, all of which are highly suggestive of a C7 radiculopathy.

(Continued)

- The presence of pathologic reflexes, including the inverted supinator, and the Hoffman and Babinski signs, are suggestive of myelopathy.
- Clonus is present and is suggestive of myelopathy.
- A Lhermitte's sign is present.
- There are no bowel and bladder signs or symptoms.
- MRI scanning is highly sensitive in the diagnosis of discogenic disease and is useful in ruling out other space-occupying lesions that may be producing radicular symptoms.
- Given the patient's age, coexistent degenerative disc disease and spondolytic changes may be contributing the patient's pain symptomatology.
- It is not uncommon for patients with cervical radiculopathy to also suffer from coexistent entrapment neuropathies, such as carpal tunnel syndrome. This is known as the double crush syndrome.
- Myelopathy is a significant finding and may require urgent surgical intervention to avoid disastrous neurologic sequalae.

Suggested Readings

Corey DL, Comeau D. Cervical radiculopathy. *Med Clin North Am.* 2014;98(4):791−799.

Leveque J-C A, Marong-Ceesay B, Cooper T, Howe CR. Diagnosis and treatment of cervical radiculopathy and myelopathy. *Phys Med Rehab Clin North Am.* 2015;26 (3):49−511.

Waldman SD. Cervical radiculopathy. *Pain Review.* 2nd ed. Philadelphia: Saunders; 2017:236−237.

Waldman SD. Functional anatomy of the cervical spine. In: *Physical Diagnosis of Pain: An Atlas of Signs and Symptoms.* 4th ed. Philadelphia: Elsevier; 2020.

Van Nguyen

A 36-year-old Male With the Inability to Feel Temperature Below the Umbilicus on the Right With Associated Upper and Lower Extremity Weakness

- Learn the common causes of cervical myelopathy.
- Learn the clinical presentation of cervical myelopathy.
- Learn how to use physical findings to identify cervical myelopathy.
- Learn how to use physical examination to determine which cervical spinal nerve roots are subserving the patient's symptoms.
- Learn to distinguish cervical myelopathy from cervical radiculopathy.
- Learn the important anatomic structures in cervical myelopathy.
- Develop an understanding of the treatment options for cervical myelopathy.
- Learn to identify red flags waving in patients who present with cervical myelopathy.
- Develop an understanding of Brown-Sequard syndrome.

Van Nguyen

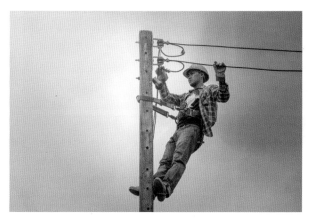

Van Nguyen is a 36 -year-old electrical lineman with a chief complaint of "when I take a shower, I can't tell if the water is too hot or too cold." "Does this occur all over your body, or is it just part of your body," I asked? Van pointed to just above his belly button on the right side and said, "It's just on the right side. . . .I really can't feel the water temperature from here on down." "Is it numb?" I asked? Van said, "You know, that's the crazy thing. . . .I can feel the water hitting me there, but I can't tell whether the water hot or cold. I can tell the water temperature on my left side, but not on the right side from my belly button on down." "Do you have any numbness or weakness anywhere else?" Van looked down and seemed reluctant to answer. He then looked at me and said, "Look, Doctor, I work as an electrical lineman for the Power and Light, and if they find out I am having problems, they won't let me work and I have two kids in college, so I really have to work." I replied that anything he told me here in the examination room stayed in the examination room, but I was really concerned that he could get himself hurt or killed if we didn't figure out what was causing his symptoms. I started again and asked, "So Van, do you have any numbness or weakness anywhere else?" He answered in a shaky voice, "Yeah, my left arm and leg are getting number and weaker. . .even though I have been taking vitamin B_{12}. . .read on the Internet that the B_{12} would help numbness." I asked Van if he was having any pain associated with his symptoms and he said, "Not really." I reassured him that we would find out what was going on; the first step was to find out exactly what was causing his symptoms.

"Van, any other symptoms I need to know about? Are you having any problems with peeing or pooping, difficulty walking, numbness, weakness, fever, chills, difficulty seeing. . .anything like that?" Van said that he didn't have any fever or chills; he could see just fine, but felt a little unsteady on his feet. He added that he had to be really careful when climbing electrical poles because he was never sure whether his left arm and leg would give out.

On physical examination, Van was afebrile and normotensive. His pulse was 76, respirations 16, and his oxygen saturation on room air was 99. Van's head, ear, eye, nose, and throat (HEENT) examination was normal, as was his

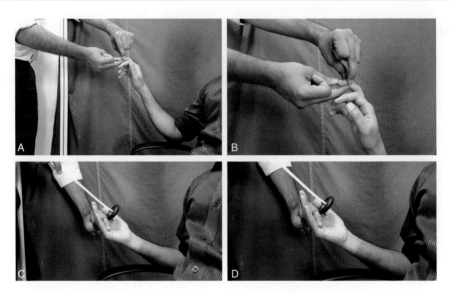

Fig. 6.1 The method of eliciting the Hoffmann and finger flexion reflexes. (A) Eliciting the Hoffman's reflex with the patient seated. The examiner stands in front of the patient. The patient's elbow rests comfortably. The wrist may be neutral or slightly palmar flexed with the forearm pronated. (B) The examiner stabilizes the middle finger just proximal to the distal interphalangeal joint. The examiner's thumb will deliver the flick to the terminal phalanx. (C) The finger flexion reflex. The elbow rests on a surface. D, The examiner places his index finger across the base of the fingers and supports the fingers with his thumb. The reflex hammer is struck onto the examiner's index finger. (From Tejus MN, Singh V, Ramesh A, et al. An evaluation of the finger flexion, Hoffman sign, and plantar reflexes as markers of cervical spinal cord compression: a comparative clinical study. *Clin Neurol Neurosurg.* 2015;134:12−16, Fig. 1.)

cardiopulmonary examination. His abdominal examination revealed no abnormal mass or organomegaly. There was no peripheral edema. He was alert and oriented. Palpation of the posterior neck muscles revealed mild tenderness to deep palpation. Range of motion of the cervical spine seemed normal. With more extreme flexion of the cervical spine, Van jumped and said that pain went down his arms, more on the left than the right. His back examination was unremarkable.

A careful neurologic examination revealed 3/5 grade left-sided weakness of the left arm and leg. There was a slight decrease in sensation of the left upper extremity. An examination of the right upper extremity revealed normal motor and sensory findings. The biceps, brachioradialis, and triceps reflexes were normal on the right, but on the left, the left biceps reflex was brisk. When I tested the left brachioradialis reflex, instead of seeing the normal reflex response of elbow flexion, I observed wrist extension, and radial wrist deviation and finger flexion consistent with an inverted supinator sign. . .really not good! The Hoffmann, finger flexion, and Babinski signs were present on the left. . . .I really wasn't liking what I was finding (Figs. 6.1 and 6.2). The right

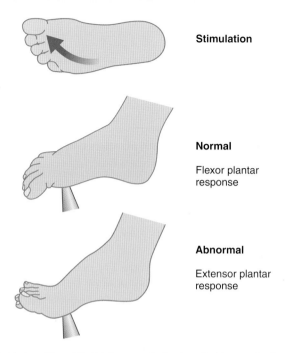

Stimulation

Normal

Flexor plantar
response

Abnormal

Extensor plantar
response

Fig. 6.2   The Babinski sign. (From Mtui E, Gruener G, Dockery P. *Fitzgerald's Clinical Neuroanatomy and Neuroscience*. 7th ed. Philadelphia: Elsevier; 2017: Fig. 16.7.)

lower extremity motor examination was normal, but the left quadriceps and Achilles reflexes were hyperactive and clonus was present bilaterally. I got Van up to walk and his gait seemed a little wobbly. I performed temperature testing with an ice cube I had obtained from the freezer in the break room and a spoon, which I warmed up under hot water from the sink. I had Van close his eyes and it was obvious that he had thermoanesthesia from about T11 down on the right. I performed a rectal examination, and both Van's anal sphincter tone and perineal sensation were normal. I told Van that I thought that something was pushing on his spinal cord and that we would need some tests to figure out what that was. Van looked really scared and asked "Doctor, is it cancer?" I answered that I really couldn't be sure and that was why the tests were so important.

Key Clinical Points—What's Important and What's Not
THE HISTORY
- No clear history of acute trauma
- No history of fever or chills

- Minimal complaints of pain
- No significant history of previous neck pain
- Unilateral thermoanesthesia on the right
- Progression of left upper and lower extremity numbness and weakness
- Neck pain with pain radiating into the upper extremity
- Feeling unsteady when walking
- No bowel or bladder symptomatology
- Worked as an electrical lineman with all attendant occupational risks

THE PHYSICAL EXAMINATION

- The patient is afebrile
- Mild tenderness of the paraspinous muscles
- Decreased sensation of the left upper and lower extremities
- Unilateral thermoanesthesia with a right T11 neurologic level
- Normal lower extremity motor examination on the right
- Pathologic reflexes present, including Hoffman's and Babinski signs, inverted supinator sign, hyperreflexia, and clonus.
- Positive Lhermitte sign (see Fig. 5.5)
- Normal anal sphincter tone

OTHER FINDINGS OF NOTE

- None

 What Tests Would You Like to Order?

The following tests were ordered:
- Magnetic resonance imaging (MRI) of the brain
- MRI of the cervical and thoracic spine
- Computer tomography (CT) of the cervical spine
- Electromyography and nerve conduction velocity testing of the left upper extremity
- Somatosensory-evoked potential testing

TEST RESULTS

Van's imaging results gave me the information that I needed to formulate a treatment plan. The good news for Van was "no cancer and no MS." The MRI of the brain revealed no plaques or tumor...it was completely normal. The CT of the cervical spine revealed a huge left-sided calcified midline herniated disc that was crushing the cervical spinal cord (Fig. 6.3). The MRI of

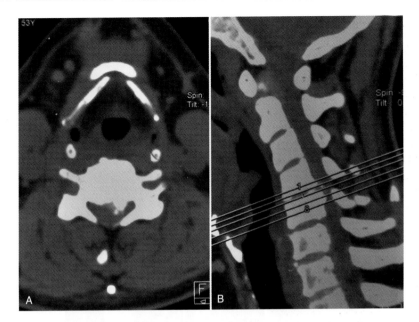

Fig. 6.3 Computed tomography (CT) of the cervical spine. Calcification of left-sided herniated C4-C5 disc (A) and posterior vertebral osteophyte of C5 (B). To deal with the osteophyte, subtotal vertebrectomy and titanium mesh cages reconstruction were selected for decompression. (From Guan D, Wang G, Clare M, Kuang Z. Brown-Sequard syndrome produced by calcified herniated cervical disc and posterior vertebral osteophyte: case report. *J Orthop.* 2015;12(suppl 2):S260–S263, Fig. 1.)

the thoracic spine was completely normal, suggesting that the lesion responsible for Van's myelopathy was the calcified disc in the cervical spine (Fig. 6.4). The MRI of the cervical spine confirmed the presence of the calcified disc at C4-C5, with a severely compromised spinal cord as indicated by the increased signal intensity on T2-weighted images (Fig. 6.5). The electromyography findings were consistent with an acute C5 radiculopathy on the left. Nerve conduction testing revealed a mild carpal tunnel on the left. Somatosensory-evoked potentials were consistent with a cervical myelopathy.

Van's myelopathy was significant and the neurosurgeon recommended immediate decompressive laminectomy. A wide decompressive laminectomy and fusion at C4-C5 was performed and the large calcified herniated cervical disc fragment was removed (Fig. 6.6). This decompressed the spinal cord and allowed it to return to a more normal position. Postoperatively, Van had to wear a rigid cervical collar. Over the next several months, Van's thermoanesthesia resolved, as did most of the numbness and weakness of his left upper and lower extremity. Van was not able to return to work climbing electrical poles, but the Power and Light found him a job as a dispatcher. All in all, a happy ending.

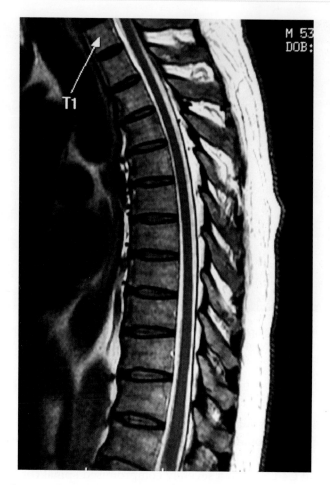

Fig. 6.4 Thoracic magnetic resonance image (MRI). No positive result indicated that the contralateral sensory disorder resulted from compression in the cervical region. (From Guan D, Wang G, Clare M, Kuang Z. Brown-Sequard syndrome produced by calcified herniated cervical disc and posterior vertebral osteophyte: Case report. *J Orthop*. 2015;12(suppl 2):S260–S263, Fig. 3.)

 Clinical Correlation—Putting It All Together

What is the diagnosis?
- Cervical myelopathy
- Brown-Sequard syndrome

The Science Behind the Diagnosis

SPINAL CORD ANATOMY

A clear understanding of the organization of the spinal cord is necessary if the clinician is to understand how pain impulses are modulated and transmitted in

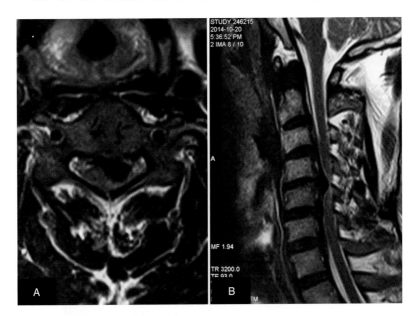

Fig. 6.5 Cervical magnetic resonance image (MRI). The herniated C4-C5 disc compressed the left side of the spinal cord (A), which is consistent with the weakness in left limb and sensory deficit in the ride side. Increased signal intensity on T2-weighted image (B) indicated severe spinal cord injury, which may lead to a poor prognosis. (From Guan D, Wang G, Clare M, Kuang Z. Brown-Sequard syndrome produced by calcified herniated cervical disc and posterior vertebral osteophyte: case report. *J Orthop.* 2015;12(suppl2):S260–S263, Fig. 2.)

health and disease. Spinal cord function can be affected by a number of diseases and the location of spinal cord damage will be directly reflected in the clinical presentation of the patient (Fig. 6.7, Box 6.1). Functionally, the spinal cord is divided in half by the anterior median fissure and the posterior median sulcus. Centrally, there is an H-shaped structure made up primarily of gray matter consisting of nerve cell bodies and glial cells (Fig. 6.8). This gray matter is pierced in its middle by the central canal. Projecting outward from the gray matter toward the points at which the dorsal and ventral roots exit the spinal cord are the horns of the gray matter. Surrounding the gray matter is the white matter, which contains the myelinated and unmyelinated axons, which are organized into tracts and columns (see Fig. 6.8).

The cell bodies of the gray matter of the spinal cord are organized into nuclei, each of which has specific functions, with the sensory nuclei grouped together in the dorsal portion of the spinal cord to receive and relay peripheral sensory information via the dorsal roots and the motor nuclei grouped together in the ventral portion of the spinal cord to relay motor commands via the ventral roots to the periphery (see Fig. 6.8). The concept that dorsal roots carry sensory information and the ventral roots carry motor information is known as the Bell-Magendie law. It should be noted that special areas of the gray matter called commissures contain axons that cross from one side of the spinal cord to the other.

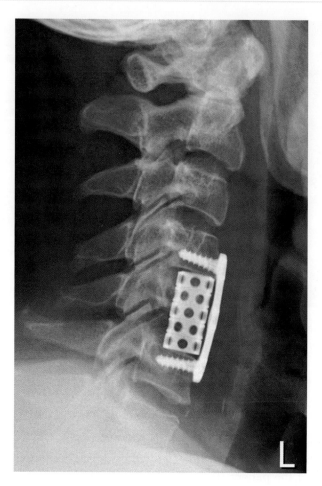

Fig. 6.6 X-ray after the operation. Subtotal vertebrectomy and titanium mesh cages reconstruction were performed through anterior approach. The cage was packed with autogenous spongy bone from removed C5 vertebra. A locking plate was implanted from C4 to C6 for stabilization (Hybrid, Stryker). (From Guan D, Wang G, Clare M, Kuang Z. Brown-Sequard syndrome produced by calcified herniated cervical disc and posterior vertebral osteophyte: case report. *J Orthop.* 2015;12(suppl 2): S260–S263, Fig. 4.)

Just as the gray matter is highly organized into nuclei, with each nucleus responsible for a specific anatomic area, the white matter is likewise organized into columns or funiculi that contain tracts, or fasciculi, whose homogeneous axons convey motor or sensory information to and from a specific anatomic area. In general, all of the axons within a tract carry information in the same direction, with the ascending tracts of white matter carrying information toward the brainstem and brain and the descending white matter tracts carrying motor commands from the higher centers into the spinal cord. Like the gray matter, there

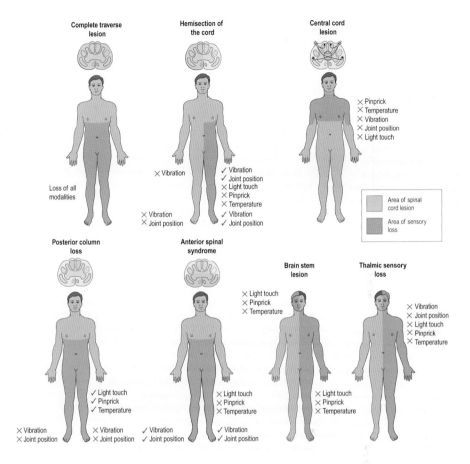

Fig. 6.7 The relationship of spinal cord lesions and clinical symptoms. (From Fuller G, Manford M. *Neurology*. 3rd ed. London: Churchill Livingstone; 2010:60—61, Fig 28.1.)

are commissural tracts within the white matter that carry sensory or motor information between spinal segments.

BROWN-SEQUARD SYNDROME

Brown-Sequard syndrome is the eponym given to the clinical picture of ipsilateral upper motor neuron paralysis and loss of proprioception combined with the loss of contralateral pain and temperature sensation (Fig. 6.9). The syndrome is caused by an incomplete spinal cord lesion characterized by the findings one would expect with hemisection of the spinal cord (see Fig. 6.9). Traumatic and nontraumatic causes of Brown-Sequard are listed in Box 6.2. Often, additional symptoms may accompany Brown-Sequard syndrome and may confuse the clinical picture. This scenario is referred to as Brown-Sequard syndrome-plus.

BOX 6.1 ■ Diseases That Affect the Spinal Cord

1. Diseases of the bony spine
2. Vascular abnormalities
3. Developmental abnormalities
   a. Hydromyelia
   b. Syringomyelia
   c. Spina bifida
   d. Diastematomyelia
4. Traumatic injury
5. Infectious and inflammatory etiology
   a. Epidural abscess
   b. Meningitis
   c. Spinal tuberculosis (Pott disease)
   d. Syphilis
   e. Mycotic infection
   f. Viral intramedullary myelitis
   g. Poliomyelitis
   h. Herpes myelitis
   i. HIV
   j. Multiple sclerosis
   k. Devic disease
   l. Idiopathic myelitis
   m. Adhesive arachnoiditis
6. Tumors
   a. Extradural primary and metastatic tumors
      i. Carcinoma, lymphoma, spinal osteoma, chordoma
   b. Intradural-extramedulary tumors
      i. Neurofibroma
      ii. Meningiomaependy
      iii. Epidermoid cysts
      iv. Demoid cyst
      v. Paraganglionma
   c. Intramedullary tumors
      i. Astrocytomas
      ii. Glioma
      iii. Oligodendroglioma
      iv. Ependymoma
      v. Hemangioblastoma
7. Nutritional and metabolic myelopathies
   a. B_{12} deficiency subacute degeneration
   b. HIV-associated vitamin deficiency
   c. Pellagra
   d. Celiac disease
   e. Lathyrism
8. Toxic myelopathies
   a. Radiation
   b. Chemical

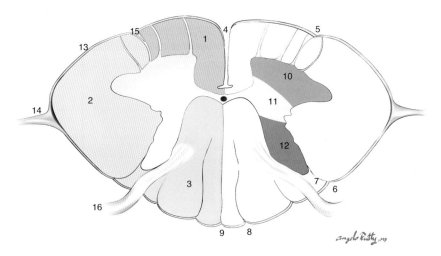

Fig. 6.8   Gross anatomy of the spinal cord in adulthood.   Representation of a transverse section of the cervical segment. 1, Anterior funicle; 2, lateral funicle; 3, posterior funicle; 4, anterior median fissure; 5, anterolateral sulcus; 6, posterolateral sulcus; 7, Lissauer's tract; 8, posterior intermediate sulcus; 9, posterior median sulcus; 10, anterior horn; 11, intermediate gray zone; 12, posterior horn; 13, pia-arachnoid; 14, denticulate ligament; 15, ventral nerve roots; 16, dorsal nerve root. (From Diaz E, Morales H. Spinal cord anatomy and clinical syndromes. *Semin Ultrasound, CT, and MRI.* 2016;37 (5):360–371, 2016: Fig 2.)

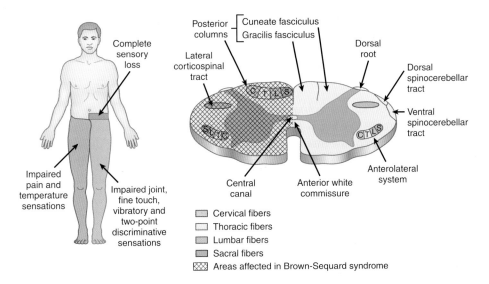

Fig. 6.9   The neuroanatomic basis of Brown-Sequard syndrome.

BOX 6.2 ■ Traumatic and Nontraumatic Causes of Brown-Sequard Syndrome

Traumatic Causes
- Stabbing
- Gunshot wound
- Motor vehicle accident
- Falls
- Surgical trauma
- Chiropractic manipulation

Nontraumatic Causes
- Cervical spondylosis
- Tumor
- Disc herniation
  - Extradural
  - Intradural
- Multiple sclerosis
- Vertebral artery dissection
- Transverse myelitis
- Ischemia
- Epidural hematoma
- Subdural hematoma
- Hematomyelia
- Epidural abscess
- Intravenous drug abuse
- Radiation
- Decompression sickness
- Spinal cord herniation
- Infection
  - Tuberculosis
  - Syphilis
  - Herpes zoster
  - Meningitis

The organization of the spinal cord explains the clinical findings of Brown-Sequard syndrome (see Fig. 6.9). The motor fibers of the corticospinal tracts decussate at the junction of the medulla and spinal cord. The ascending dorsal column, which carries vibration and position information, runs ipsilateral to the roots of entry and crosses above the spinal cord in the medulla. The spinothalamic tracts carry pain, temperature, and crude touch sensations from the contralateral side of the body. At the site of spinal cord injury, nerve roots and/or anterior horn cells also may be affected, leading to Brown-Sequard syndrome-plus.

CERVICAL MYELOPATHY

Cervical radiculopathy and myelopathy can exist independently or can coexist. In some patients, the signs and symptoms of cervical radiculopathy are obvious,

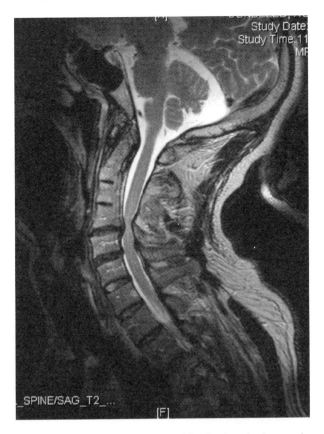

Fig. 6.10 Cervical spondylotic myelopathy. T2-weighted spin-echo image, demonstrating compression of the spinal cord at multiple levels resulting in grossly narrowed cervical spinal canal, with mild hyperintensity of the spinal cord at the level of compression, caused by myelomalacia. (From Schapira A. *Neurology and Clinical Neuroscience*. Philadelphia: Mosby; 2007: Fig. 40.5.)

and the signs and symptoms of myelopathy are extremely subtle. The converse can also be true. Because of the devastating impact that cervical myelopathy can have on the patient, it must be a diagnostic consideration in any patient who presents with neck pain, radiculopathy, or any symptoms suggestive of spinal cord compromise.

Cervical spondylotic myelopathy is a common degenerative condition of the cervical spine and is the most common cause of nontraumatic myelopathy in older adults (Fig. 6.10). In most instances, cervical spondylitic myelopathy is the end result of degenerative disc disease. As the cervical intervertebral discs age, mechanical stresses are placed on the cervical spine. These stresses produce osteophytes, which can impinge on nerve roots and compress the spinal cord. Associated facet arthropathy and hypertrophy of the ligamentum flavum can further contribute the evolution of cervical spondylotic myelopathy.

Cervical spondylotic myelopathy usually develops insidiously, unless there is acute trauma to the cervical spine and its contents. Early symptoms may include neck pain and stiffness. Radicular pain and shock like paresthesias into the upper extremities may also develop. Often, multiple spinal segments are affected with patients suffering from a high compressive myelopathy (C3-C5), often complaining of neck pain and stiffness with associated hand clumsiness and numbness. When this occurs, patients will often describe difficulty in writing, dropping things, a loss of manual dexterity (e.g., inability to button a shirt or fasten a bra, and a sense that their hands "are not working right.") Patients with a lower myelopathy typically present with weakness, stiffness, and difficulty in walking, especially in the dark, owing to loss of proprioception in the lower extremities. These patients often exhibit signs of spasticity and hyperreflexia as well as pathologic reflexes (e.g., Babinski sign, clonus), which will often be identified on physical examination. Urinary and bowel incontinence are less common, but difficult fully emptying the bladder with associated frequency and hesitancy is often seen.

In patients with preexisting cervical spondylosis, acute trauma to the cervical spine, most commonly acute hyperextension injuries from motor vehicle accidents, can result in an acute cervical myelopathy. In this setting, there is often greater upper extremity weakness than lower extremity weakness, varying degrees of sensory disturbances below the lesion, and the rapid evolution of myelopathic findings, such as spasticity and urinary retention.

The concept of diagnosing a problem at a specific neurologic level via physical examination has its basis in the fact that pathology at the cervical spinal cord or cervical nerve root level manifests itself in a relatively consistent manner by dysfunction, numbness, and pain of the upper extremity, which occurs in a dermatomal distribution. Although not foolproof, a careful physical examination of the upper extremity with an eye to the neurologic level affected can frequently guide the clinician in designing a more targeted workup and treatment plan. By overlapping the information gleaned from physical examination with the neuroanatomic information gained from magnetic resonance imaging and the neurophysiologic information from electromyography, a highly accurate diagnosis can be made as to which level of the cervical spine is responsible for the patient's symptoms.

MANAGEMENT AND TREATMENT

The presence of physical findings of cervical myelopathy are strong indications for surgical intervention (e.g., decompressive laminectomy, anterior cervical fusion and discectomy). Relative indications for surgical intervention include progressive neurologic deficit, recurrent radiculopathy, persistent radiculopathy, and/or severe axial neck pain that has failed to respond to aggressive conservative therapy. The more acute and severe the myelopathy, the more urgent the need for decompression of the cervical spinal cord. High-dose intravenous steroids may reduce spinal cord swelling and also may decrease the extent of permanent neurologic deficit. The clinician must always be cognizant of the fact that more than one pathologic process may be responsible for the patient's symptomatology and compromise of the spinal cord may occur at more than one level (see Fig. 6.10).

HIGH-YIELD TAKEAWAYS

- The patient is afebrile, making an acute infectious etiology (e.g., epidural abscess) unlikely.
- The patient's neurologic examination is grossly abnormal, with ipsilateral numbness and weakness and contralateral thermoanesthesia.
- Pathologic reflexes, including the inverted supinator, Hoffman, finger flexion, and Babinski signs are highly abnormal and suggestive of myelopathy.
- Clonus is present and is suggestive of myelopathy.
- A Lhermitte sign is present.
- There are no bowel or bladder symptoms.
- MRI scanning is highly sensitive in the diagnosis of discogenic disease and is useful in ruling out other space-occupying lesions that may be producing radicular symptoms.
- Given the patient's age, coexistent degenerative disc disease and spondylotic changes may be contributing the patient's pain symptomatology.
- It is not uncommon for patients with cervical radiculopathy also to suffer from coexistent entrapment neuropathies, such as carpal tunnel syndrome. This is known as the double crush syndrome.
- Myelopathy is a significant finding and may require urgent surgical intervention to avoid disastrous neurologic sequalae.

Suggested Readings

Akter F, Kotter M. Pathobiology of degenerative cervical myelopathy. *Neurosurg Clin North Am.* 2018;29(1):13–19.

Badhiwala JH, Wilson JR. The natural history of degenerative cervical myelopathy. *Neurosurg Clin North Am.* 2018;29(1):21–32.

Corey DL, Comeau D. Cervical radiculopathy. *Med Clin North Am.* 2014;98(4):791–799.

Leveque J-CA, Marong-Ceesay B, Cooper T, Howe CR. Diagnosis and treatment of cervical radiculopathy and myelopathy. *Phys Med Rehabil Clin North Am.* 2015;26 (3):491–522.

Waldman SD. Cervical radiculopathy. In: *Pain Review.* 2nd ed. Philadelphia: Saunders; 2017:236–237.

Waldman SD. Functional anatomy of the cervical spine. In: *Physical Diagnosis of Pain: An Atlas of Signs and Symptoms.* 4th ed. Philadelphia: Elsevier; 2020.

Elsa Hartvigsen

An 89-Year-Old Female With
Sharp Pain Between the
Shoulder Blades

- Learn the common causes of thoracic vertebral compression fractures.
- Learn the clinical presentation of thoracic vertebral compression fractures.
- Learn how to use physical examination to determine which thoracic spinal nerve root is compromised by a vertebral compression fracture.
- Learn to distinguish thoracic vertebral fracture from other causes of thoracic pain.
- Learn the important anatomic structures affected by vertebral fracture.
- Develop an understanding of the significant morbidity and mortality associated with vertebral compression fracture.
- Understand which specific patient populations are most at risk for vertebral compression fracture.
- Develop an understanding of the treatment options for vertebral compression fracture.
- Learn to identify red flags waving in patients who present with acute thoracic vertebral compression fracture.
- Develop an understanding of the role in interventional pain management in the treatment of thoracic vertebral compression fracture.
- Understand the importance of early identification and treatment of osteoporosis.

Elsa Hartvigsen

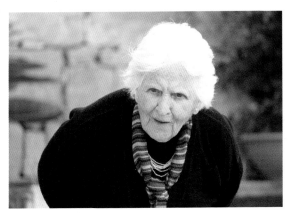

Elsa Hartvigsen is an 89-year-old woman with a chief complaint of sharp pain between the shoulder blades. Elsa went on to say that it hurt so much, that the pain knocked her to the ground. "Doctor, the pain was worse than when I had that kidney stone. I knew I couldn't just lie there on the ground for all of the neighbors to see … so I gathered up my strength and tried to get up, but it hurt too much…so I crawled back into the house on my hands and knees and called out for Betty…she came helped me get back into bed…she is such a gem."

In reviewing Elsa's chart, I was struck by the fact that over the years, Elsa had been amazingly healthy. She was on no prescription medications and had never been hospitalized. She had had a hysterectomy and bilateral oophorectomy in the very distant past for dysfunctional uterine bleeding and had never been on any hormone replacement therapy since her hysterectomy. Over the years, Elsa's Pap smears and mammograms were all normal and she was current on all of her immunizations. Looking at her lying there in pain, I had a pretty good idea what was wrong and it suddenly hit me that I had really dropped the ball on this one. Elsa was always so vibrant, fit, efficient, positive, and healthy that I had failed to take measures to prevent or at least forestall what had surely happened to her.

I asked Elsa to tell me exactly where the pain was and she said it was "right in the middle of my back." She went on to say that when she moved, it got worse and that the pain would shoot out into her kidneys. I asked her what made it better and she volunteered that she had "tried Extra Strength Tylenol, a heating pad, and analgesic balm," none of which really helped. She said, "It does feel better when Betty rubs the area where it hurts." She admitted that getting up to the commode had just about killed her, but she was not about to make Betty empty a bedpan. She denied any bowel or bladder symptomatology related to her pain. Betty said that even though it really hurt, Elsa insisted on getting out of bed and getting dressed to come to her appointment with me. But when Elsa bent over to try and get into Betty's Prius, it hurt so bad that she had to give up and go back to bed.

I told Elsa that I was going to look her over and that we would get her back to normal as soon as possible. She sighed heavily and said, "You are my doctor and I trust you with my life...but please don't make promises you can't keep!" I reassured her and with great difficulty, helped her sit up on the side of her bed. She sat bent forward and was in obvious pain. Examination of her thoracic spine revealed Elsa was a lot more kyphotic than I remembered. There was moderate spasm of the thoracic paraspinous muscles bilaterally. No rash was present. Pain was elicited on flexion of the thoracic spine, with some relief of pain on extension. There was no costo-vertebral angle tenderness to percussion. Her upper motor and sensory examination was normal, as was her lower extremity motor and sensory examination. Deep tendon reflexes were physiologic throughout and no pathologic reflexes were identified. Elsa's head, ears, eyes, nose, and throat (HEENT) examination was grossly normal and her cardiopulmonary exami-nation was unremarkable. The abdominal examination was bland, with nor-mal bowel sounds. There was no peripheral edema.

I told Elsa what I thought was wrong and why she was having so much pain. I also told her that I wanted to order some x-rays and laboratory tests to confirm the diagnosis and make sure nothing else was going on. Elsa immediately protested that she couldn't get into Betty's car and I reassured her that I would have a wheelchair van pick her up and take her to the hos-pital outpatient department for the tests so she wouldn't have to get into Betty's Prius. Elsa started to object to the idea of a wheelchair, but then resignedly sighed and said, "You are my doctor and I trust you to do what's right." I called in a prescription for a few lidocaine patches and a small amount of hydrocodone with acetaminophen. I told her not to get up by her-self if she took the pain pills because they could make her dizzy and I didn't want to have to sew up her head if she fell. Elsa took my hand in both of hers and with great feeling, said, "You are my doctor and I know you will take care of me....so don't you be worried about me. I will do everything you tell me to do." I arranged for wheelchair van transport for Elsa to the hospital outpatient department for testing.

Key Clinical Points—What's Important and What's Not
THE HISTORY

- History of the sudden onset of thoracic spine pain after seemingly trivial trauma
- No significant history of previous thoracic spine pain or other pain complaints
- The presence of pain that radiated bilaterally from the mid-thoracic spine anteriorly

- A distant history of renal calculi
- No bowel or bladder symptomatology
- Surgically induced menopause in the distant past

THE PHYSICAL EXAMINATION

- The patient is afebrile
- Dorsal kyphosis
- Spasm of thoracic paraspinous muscles in the area of maximal pain
- Normal neurologic examination
- No pathologic reflexes
- No rash
- Normal cardiopulmonary examination
- Normal abdominal examination
- No costovertebral angle tenderness to percussion

OTHER FINDINGS OF NOTE

- None

 What Tests Would You Like to Order?

The following tests were ordered:
- Plain radiographs of the thoracic spine
- Computed tomography (CT) of the thoracic spine
- Dual-energy x-ray absorptiometry (DEXA) scan
- Magnetic resonance imaging (MRI) of the thoracic spine
- Complete blood count (CBC)
- Urinalysis
- Comprehensive metabolic panel (CMP)
- Serum protein electrophoresis
- Electrocardiogram (ECG)

TEST RESULTS

Elsa's urinalysis, CBC, CPM, serum protein electrophoresis, and ECG were all normal. Her imaging studies were a mess. Plain radiographs of the thoracic spine revealed multiple vertebral compression fractures and degenerative changes (Fig. 7.1). Elsa's DEXA scan revealed severe osteoporosis (Fig. 7.2). Her MRI scan revealed both acute and chronic vertebral compression fractures (Fig. 7.3). Her CT scan confirmed these findings.

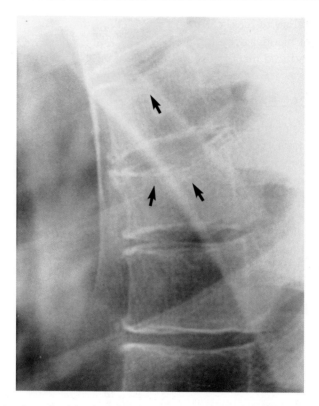

Fig. 7.1   Lateral radiograph of the thoracic spine demonstrates anterior wedge-shaped compression fractures of the fourth and fifth thoracic vertebral bodies. Observe the anterior and central endplate depressions (*arrows*). (From Taylor J, Hughes T, Resnick D. *Skeletal Imaging*. 2nd ed. Maryland Heights: Saunders; 2010: Fig. 3.25.)

 Clinical Correlation—Putting It All Together

What is the diagnosis?
- Acute vertebral compression fracture

The Science Behind the Diagnosis

Thoracic vertebral compression fracture is one of the most common causes of thoracic spine pain. Osteoporosis is the leading cause of thoracic vertebral compression fractures (Fig. 7.4). Thoracic vertebral compression fractures are also associated with trauma to the dorsal spine owing to acceleration/deceleration injuries. Rarely, tumors or infection involving the thoracic vertebrae as well as other causes of osteopenia, including hyperparathyroidism, may result in vertebral compression fracture (Box 7.1). In patients with osteoporosis or in those

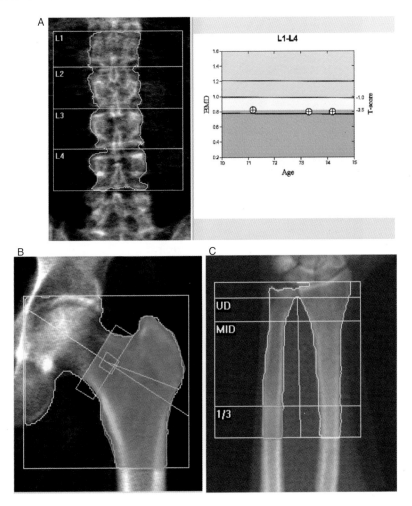

Fig. 7.2 (A) Dual-energy x-ray absorptiometry (DEXA) study of the lumbar spine. (B) The proximal femur and the distal radius (C) obtained in an elderly woman with osteoporotic bone mineral density (BMD). The diagnosis is made using the lowest t score from L1—4, femoral neck, total femur (consists of femoral neck, trochanteric, and intertrochanteric region, shown in blue), and one third distal radius regions (shown in blue). In this patient, the t score of the lumbar spine was −2.7, of the neck −2.7, of the total femur −2.4, and of the one third distal radius region −2.6. (From Link TM. Radiology of osteoporosis. *Can Assoc Radiol J* 2016;67(1):28−40, Fig. 7.)

with primary tumors or metastatic disease involving the thoracic vertebrae, the fracture may occur with coughing (tussive fractures) or spontaneously.

The pain and functional disability associated with fractures of the vertebrae are determined in large part by the severity of injury (e.g., the number of vertebrae involved) and the nature of the injury (e.g., whether the fracture creates spinal instability allowing impingement on the spinal nerves or the spinal cord

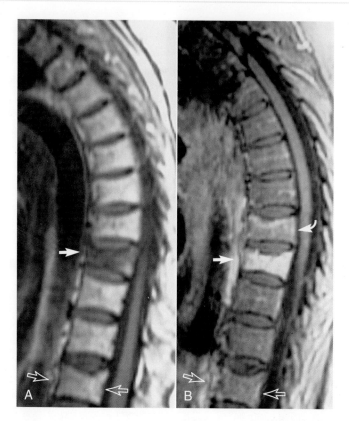

Fig. 7.3 Acute compression fracture: magnetic resonance imaging (MRI) abnormalities. (A and B) A 63--year-old woman with severe kyphosis and acute thoracic spinal pain. Sagittal T1-weighted spin echo MRI obtained before (TR/TE, 500/12) (A) and after (TR/TE, 800/12) (B) intravenous administration of gadolinium contrast agent reveal a wedge-shaped compression deformity of T10 vertebral body *(arrow)*. Low-signal intensity is seen in the pregadolinium image (A) and high-signal intensity in the postgadolinium image (B), which is characteristic of a recently fractured vertebra. Compare the findings of the acute fracture in T10 with those of a remote, healed fracture of L1 *(open arrows)*. In the remote fracture, the signal intensity of the L1 vertebral body is the same as that of the adjacent vertebral bodies before (A) and after (B) contrast agent administration. A subacute fracture of T9 also is evident *(curved arrow)*, in which the signal is less intense than that of the acute fracture on the postgadolinium image (B). Note high-signal intensity in the prevertebral soft tissues in (B). Compression fractures are common, especially in older women. MRI can be useful in differentiating between recent (acute) and long-standing (chronic) spine fractures and is well suited for assessing spinal cord and soft tissue injury. However, differentiating between benign compression fractures and neoplastic, pathologic fractures can be difficult. The finding on MRI of a fluid collection within a collapsed vertebral body may represent osteonecrosis secondary to vertebral collapse. (From Taylor J, Hughes T, Resnick D. *Skeletal Imaging*. 2nd ed. Maryland Heights: Saunders; 2010: Fig. 3.28.)

itself). The severity of pain associated with thoracic vertebral compression fracture may range from a dull, deep ache with minimal compression of the vertebrae without nerve impingement to severe sharp, stabbing pain that limits the patient's ability to ambulate and cough.

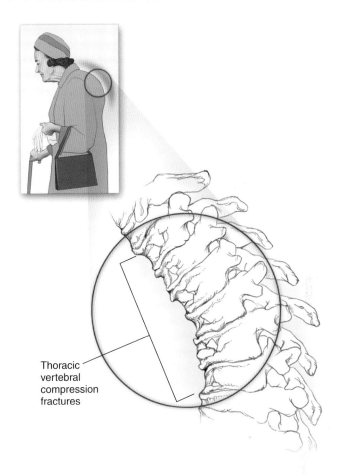

Fig. 7.4 Osteoporosis is a common cause of thoracic vertebral fractures. (From Waldman SD. *Atlas of Common Pain Syndromes* 4th ed. Philadelphia: Elsevier; 2019: Fig. 73.1.)

BOX 7.1 ■ Differential Diagnosis of Vertebral Compression Fracture

- Pathologic fractures secondary to bone metastases from cancer
- Leukemia
- Lymphoma
- Metastatic disease
- Multiple myeloma
- Hyperparathyroidism
- Paget disease
- Scurvy
- Renal osteodystrophy
- Sickle cell anemia
- Homocystinuria/homocysteinemia

SIGNS AND SYMPTOMS

Compression fractures of the thoracic vertebrae are aggravated by deep inspiration, coughing, and any movement of the thoracic spine. Palpation of the affected vertebrae may elicit pain and reflex spasm of the paraspinous musculature of the dorsal spine. If trauma has occurred, hematoma and ecchymosis overlying the fracture site may be present. If trauma has occurred, the clinician should be aware of the possibility of damage to the bony thorax and the intraabdominal and intrathoracic contents. If the compression fracture compromises the spinal canal, myelopathy may result (Fig. 7.5). Damage to the spinal nerves from collapse of the lateral portion of the vertebra may produce abdominal ileus and severe pain, with resulting splinting of the paraspinous muscles of the dorsal spine further compromising the patient's ability to walk and his or her pulmonary status (Fig. 7.6). Failure to treat this pain and splinting aggressively may result in a negative cycle of hypoventilation, atelectasis, and ultimately pneumonia.

TESTING

Plain radiographs of the vertebrae are indicated in all patients who present with pain from thoracic vertebral compression fracture to rule out other

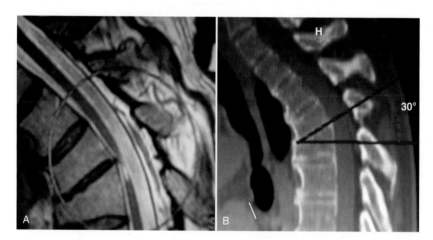

Fig. 7.5 (A) T2-weighted magnetic resonance image (MRI) sequence sagittal view, showing the ventral spinal cord compression and stretching resulting from the posttraumatic focal kyphosis at the level of T4. At the T4 level, the spinal cord is markedly atrophied and shows a significantly increased signal, consistent with spinal cord injury. (B) Sagittal thoracic computed tomography (CT) scan showing a healed compression fracture at T4, the level with a resultant focal kyphosis of approximately 30 degrees. (From Yue J, Guyer R, Johnson JP, Khoo L, Hochschuler S. *The Comprehensive Treatment of the Aging Spine*. Philadelphia: Saunders; 2010: Fig. 45.4.)

occult fractures and other bony pathology, including tumor (see Fig. 7.1). With a history of trauma or a suspicion of malignancy, radionuclide bone scanning may be useful to rule out occult fractures of the vertebrae as well as primary or metastatic tumors involving the spine. With no history of trauma, bone density testing to rule out osteoporosis is appropriate, as are serum protein electrophoresis and testing for hyperparathyroidism (see Fig. 7.2). Based on the patient's clinical presentation, additional testing, including complete blood count, prostate-specific antigen, erythrocyte sedimentation rate, and antinuclear antibody testing, may be indicated. Computed tomography scan of the thoracic contents is indicated if occult mass or significant trauma to the thoracic contents is suspected (Fig. 7.7). Electrocardiogram to rule out cardiac contusion is indicated in all patients with traumatic sternal fractures or with significant anterior dorsal spine trauma. MRI of the spine is also useful in helping distinguish between acute

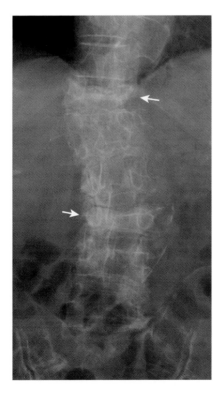

Fig. 7.6 **Anteroposterior radiograph of an elderly woman with osteoporosis.** Scoliosis is present, as well as vertebral compression factures that are more prominent on the concave aspects of the scoliosis at T11 and L3 (*white arrows*). The lateral compression fractures coexist with anterior wedge fractures and may be the result of scoliosis rather than its cause. (From Waldman SD, Campbell RSD. *Imaging of Pain*. Philadelphia: Saunders; 2011: Fig. 28.2.)

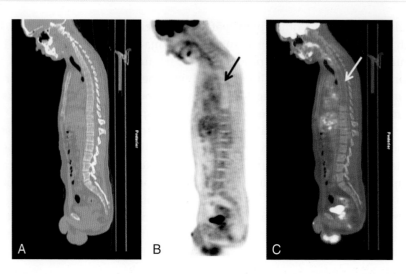

Fig. 7.7 Vertebral compression fractures. A–C, Sagittal computed tomography (CT), FDG-PET, and fused PET/CT images showing decreased FDG marrow uptake in thoracic vertebrae following external beam radiation for mediastinal malignancy (*arrows* in B, C). FDG-PET, Fluorodeoxyglucose-positron emission tomography. (From Waldman, SD. *Atlas of Common Pain Syndromes*. 4th ed. Philadelphia: Elsevier; 2019: Fig. 73.3.)

and chronic vertebral insufficiency fractures as well as identifying pathologic vertebral fractures and other abnormalities not identified on other imaging modalities (Fig. 7.8).

DIFFERENTIAL DIAGNOSIS

Usually the diagnosis of thoracic vertebral compression fracture is easily made in the setting of trauma. In the setting of spontaneous vertebral fracture secondary to osteoporosis or metastatic disease, the diagnosis may be confusing. In this setting, the pain of occult rib fracture is often mistaken for pain of cardiac or gallbladder origin and can lead to visits to the emergency department and unnecessary cardiac and gastrointestinal workups. Acute sprain of the thoracic paraspinous muscles can be confused with thoracic vertebral compression fracture, especially if the patient has been coughing. Because the pain of acute herpes zoster may precede the rash by 24 to 72 hours, the pain may be erroneously attributed to vertebral compression fracture (Fig. 7.9).

MANAGEMENT AND TREATMENT

Initial treatment of pain secondary to compression fracture of the thoracic spine should include a combination of simple analgesics and nonsteroidal anti-

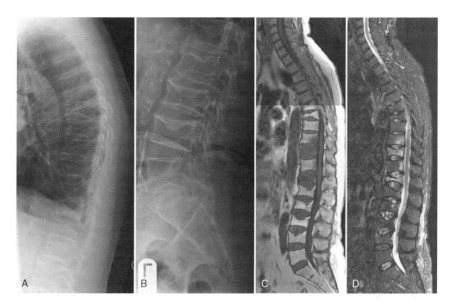

Fig. 7.8   Lateral radiographs of the thoracic (A) and lumbar (B) spine demonstrate multilevel anterior vertebral body fractures. It is not possible to distinguish between acute and chronic fractures. The sagittal T1-weighted (C) and short tau inversion recovery (STIR) (D) magnetic resonance images (MRI), however, visualize multiple anterior wedge fractures. The recent acute fractures have marrow edema, which are low signal intensity (SI) on the T1-weighted MRI and high SI on the STIR image. The chronic fractures have normal fatty marrow SI. (From Waldman SD. *Atlas of Common Pain Syndromes*. 4th ed. Philadelphia: Elsevier; 2019: Fig. 73.2.)

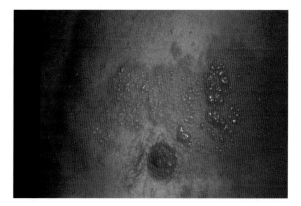

Fig. 7.9   The pain of acute herpes zoster may mimic the pain of vertebral compression fracture. It is important to remember that the pain of acute herpes zoster may begin a few days before the vesicular rash appears.

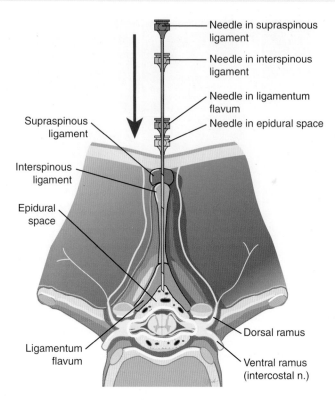

Fig. 7.10 Thoracic epidural block. When performing a thoracic epidural block in the midline, pass the needle through several structures. After traversing the skin and subcutaneous tissues, the styletted epidural needle impinges on the supraspinous ligament, which runs vertically between the apices of the spinous processes. The interspinous ligament, which runs obliquely between the spinous processes, is encountered next, offering additional resistance to needle advancement. Because the interspinous ligament is contiguous with the ligamentum flavum, the pain management specialist may perceive a false loss of resistance when the needle tip enters the space between the interspinous ligament and the ligamentum flavum. *n.*, Nerve. (From Waldman SD. *Atlas of Interventional Pain Management*. 4th ed. Philadelphia: Saunders; 2015: Fig. 63.4.)

inflammatory agents or the cyclooxygenase-2 inhibitors. If these medications do not control the patient's symptomatology adequately, short-acting potent opioid analgesics, such as hydrocodone, represent a reasonable next step. As the opioid analgesics have the potential to suppress the cough reflex and respiration, the clinician must be careful to monitor the patient closely and to instruct the patient in adequate pulmonary toilet techniques.

The local application of heat and cold may also be beneficial to provide symptomatic relief of the pain of vertebral fracture. The use of an orthotic (e.g., the Cash brace) may also help provide symptomatic relief. For patients who do not respond to these treatment modalities, thoracic epidural block with local anesthetic and steroid is a reasonable next step (Fig. 7.10). Ongoing treatment of

---

BOX 7.2 ■ Pharmacologic Treatments for Osteoporosis

Bisphosphonates
- Ibandronate (Boniva)
- Alendronate (Binosto, Fosamax)
- Risedronate (Actonel, Atelvia)
- Zoledronic acid (Reclast, Zometa)

Monoclonal antibody medications
- Denosumab (Prolia, Xgeva)

Hormone-related therapy
- Estrogen
- Raloxifene (Evista)
- Testosterone (in men)

Bone-building medications
- Romosozumab (Evenity)
- Teriparatide (Forteo)
- Abaloparatide (Tymlos)

---

underlying osteoporosis is important to preclude, or at least delay, the progression of the osteoporosis. Box 7.2 lists the pharmacologic treatments available for osteoporosis.

HIGH-YIELD TAKEAWAYS

- The patient is afebrile, making an acute infectious etiology such as infection of adjacent structures, e.g., Pott disease or discitis or epidural abscess unlikely.
- The patient's symptomatology is the result of seemingly minor trauma to the thoracic spine.
- The patient has a remote history of surgical menopause.
- The patient has dorsal kyphosis.
- The patient's pain is localized in the midthoracic spine and radiates anteriorly.
- The patient's pain is made worse with flexion of the thoracic spine.
- There was no rash suggestive of acute herpes zoster.
- The urinalysis was negative, making the diagnosis of renal calculi unlikely.
- There were no elevated calcium levels on the CMP, making hyperparathyroidism unlikely.
- The serum protein electrophoresis was normal, making multiple myeloma unlikely.

(Continued)

- The patient's symptoms are bilateral.
- The patient's neurologic examination was normal.
- There are no bowel or bladder symptoms or pathologic reflexes suggestive of myelopathy.
- MRI of the spine is highly sensitive in the diagnosis of spinal cord compression and is useful in ruling out other space-occupying lesions that may be producing radicular symptoms (e.g., primary or metastatic tumor, epidural abscess, hematoma).
- MRI of the spine is also useful in both helping distinguish between acute and chronic vertebral insufficiency fractures and identifying pathologic vertebral fractures.
- CT scanning useful in the diagnosis of bony abnormalities of the spine and is helpful in characterizing the nature of vertebral compression fractures.
- CT scanning may be useful in assessing the stability of vertebral fractures.
- Given the patient's age, coexistent degenerative disc disease and spondylotic changes may be contributing the patient's pain symptomatology.
- Other diseases may cause vertebral compression fractures (see Box 7.1).

Suggested Readings

Waldman SD. Functional anatomy of the thoracic spine. In: *Physical Diagnosis of Pain: An Atlas of Signs and Symptoms*. 4th ed. Philadelphia: Elsevier; 2020.

Waldman SD. Thoracic epidural nerve block: The translaminar approach. In: *Atlas of Interventional Pain Management*. 5th ed. Philadelphia: Elsevier; 2020.

Waldman SD. Thoracic radiculopathy. In: *Pain Review*. 2nd ed. Philadelphia: Saunders; 2017:228—229.

Goz V, Errico TJ, Weinreb JH, et al. Vertebroplasty and kyphoplasty: national outcomes and trends in utilization from 2005 through 2010. *Spine J*. 2015;15(5):959—965.

Kendler L, Bauer DC, Davison KS, et al. Vertebral fractures: clinical importance and management. *Am J Med*. 2016;129(2):e1-221.e10.

Miller PD. Clinical management of vertebral compression fractures. *J Clin Densitom*. 2016;19(1):97—101.

Schousboe JT. Epidemiology of vertebral fractures. *J Clin Densitom*. 2016;19(1):8—22.

Waldman SD. Percutaneous kyphoplasty. In: *Atlas of Interventional Pain Management*. 4th ed. Philadelphia: Elsevier; 2016:866—873.

Waldman SD. Percutaneous vertebroplasty. In: *Atlas of Interventional Pain Management*. 4th ed. Philadelphia: Elsevier; 2016:874—878.

CHAPTER

8

Cam Johnson

A 15-Year-Old Female With Severe Back Pain and an Inability to Walk

LEARNING OBJECTIVES

- Learn the common causes of epidural abscess.
- Learn the risk factors associated with epidural abscess.
- Learn the clinical presentation of epidural abscess.
- Learn the classic triad.
- Learn how to use physical findings to identify neurologic compromise associated with epidural abscess.
- Learn how to use physical findings to determine the level of spinal cord compromise from epidural abscess.
- Learn to distinguish epidural abscess from other causes of myelopathy.
- Learn the important anatomic structures involved in epidural abscess.
- Develop an understanding of the treatment options for epidural abscess.
- Learn to identify red flags waving in patients who present with epidural abscess.

Cam Johnson

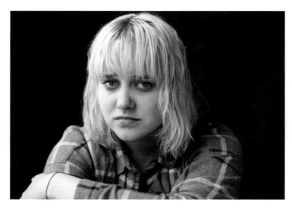

Cam Johnson is a 15-year-old female with a chief complaint of "There is something friggin' wrong with my legs." Cam was homeless and found unconscious behind a dumpster and brought to the emergency room. Narcan was administered en route to the emergency room and the patient became alert and agitated, demanding to be let out of the ambulance.

"Cam, the nurse says you are really sick. Do you know where you are?" "Yeah, I'm at University Hospital and I need to get the hell out of here." She struggled to get up, but didn't have the strength, so she flopped back down in bed. She said, "Doctor, can I get something for the pain? My back is really killing me!" I told her we needed to wait until we figured out what was going on. She said, "There is something really, really wrong with my legs. I can't walk and it's freezing in here." I looked at her vitals and her temperature was 103.4. She was normotensive, but tachycardic and breathing about 24 times a minute. Her oxygen saturation was 95 on room air.

I asked Cam when the problem with her legs started and she said that she thought it was about 2 or 3 days ago. She thought she just had the flu. She said she was having trouble keeping anything down and again asked for something to treat the pain. "Tell me where the pain is," I asked. She said, "It's right in the middle of my back. My legs really hurt and I can't walk. I think I peed in my pants." I told her that once we figured out what was wrong, we would get her all cleaned up. She again said that she needed to get out of here.

I asked Cam if it was OK for me to examine her and she shrugged and said "Whatever." I examined her head for signs of trauma. There were a couple of old scars, but nothing acute. Her sclerae were icteric and on fundoscopic examination, I saw Roth spots (Fig. 8.1). I took a quick look at her nails and immediately identified splinter hemorrhages (Fig. 8.2). Her arms were black and blue and it was obvious she had been shooting up. I asked Cam what drugs she was using and she said, "Whatever I can get." "So what were you shooting up today?" I asked. Cam shrugged and answered "Crushed-up Oxy. . .Hey, Doc, I really need something for the pain." I said I would get her something as soon as my colleague, who was a specialist in nonmoving legs, saw her. I listened to her heart

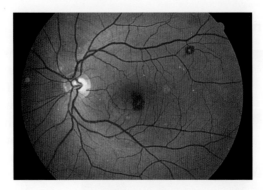

Fig. 8.1   Roth spots. (From Goldman L, Schafer A. *Goldman's Cecil Medicine*. 24th ed. Philadelphia: Saunders; 2012: Fig. 431.28.)

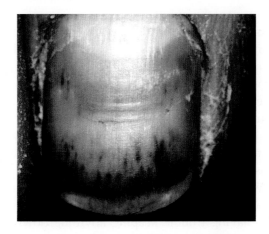

Fig. 8.2   Splinter hemorrhages beneath the nail are often seen in infectious endocarditis. (From Saladi RN, Persaud AN, Rudikoff D, Cohen SR. Idiopathic splinter hemorrhages. *J Am Acad Dermatol.* 2004; (2):289−292, Fig. 2.)

and she had a loud tricuspid murmur. Cam had severe pain to percussion of the lower thoracic spine with associated spasm of the lower thoracic paraspinous muscles. Her liver was enlarged and I could feel the tip of her spleen. Her dentition was terrible, as was her breath.

Cam's upper extremity motor and sensory examination was normal and her deep tendon reflexes were physiologic. Cam had a sensory level of about T11 with almost complete anesthesia on the right and impaired sensation on the left. Her lower extremity examination revealed only a trace of motor function bilaterally. Babinski sign was present bilaterally. Rectal examination revealed decreased rectal sphincter tone and decreased perineal sensation.

I said to Cam, "I want you to listen to me very carefully because this is really serious...you have something pressing on your spinal cord, which is why your legs won't work and why you are having all this pain and numbness. I need to take you to surgery immediately if we are to have any hope of getting you better." Cam said, "I don't want any surgery...I want to get out of here." I took Cam's hand and looked her straight in the eye. "Cam, you need to listen to me...you really need to do what I say or you will probably be paralyzed and will probably die." I squeezed her hand and said, "I promise you that I will be here when you get out of surgery and together, we will figure this out...I will take care of you...you know you can count on me." Cam looked away, shrugged, and said, "Whatever." Her shrug seemed to conveyed her complete and utter despair. "Are you ready to go to surgery?" Cam whispered, "Yes...please help me."

Key Clinical Points—What's Important and What's Not

THE HISTORY

- No clear history of acute spinal trauma
- History of IV drug abuse
- History of homelessness
- History of flu like illness
- History of fever and chills
- History of severe mid-back pain
- History of difficulty walking
- History of urinary incontinence
- Progression of left upper and lower extremity numbness and weakness
- No upper extremity symptoms

THE PHYSICAL EXAMINATION

- The patient is febrile
- The patient has chills
- Bruising and ecchymosis suggestive of repeated IV drug abuse
- The patient may be in acute opioid withdrawal following administration of naloxone by the emergency medical technicians (EMTs)
- Spasm of the thoracic paraspinous muscles
- Pain elicited to percussion of the lower thoracic spine
- Significant weakness of the lower extremities
- T11 incomplete sensory level
- Babinski sign present bilaterally

- Roth spots on the retina (see Fig. 8.1)
- Subungual splinter hemorrhages (see Fig. 8.2)
- Tricuspid murmur
- Decreased anal sphincter tone
- Decreased sensation of the perineum

OTHER FINDINGS OF NOTE

- Depressive affect

 ## What Tests Would You Like to Order?

The following tests were ordered:
- Blood cultures
- Magnetic resonance imaging (MRI) of the thoracic and lumbar spine
- Complete blood count
- Erythrocyte sedimentation rate
- Hepatitis panel
- HIV test
- Comprehensive metabolic profile

TEST RESULTS

Cam's imaging results gave us the information we needed to formulate a treatment plan. Cam was desperately ill with sepsis and a T11 paraparesis. She had significant spinal cord compromise, but there was some hope that we could improve her neurologic status with surgical intervention. An MRI scan of her thoracic spine revealed a large epidural abscess with associated vertebral osteomyelitis and discitis (Fig. 8.3). Her complete blood count revealed mild anemia with immature cells and a white count of 14,800 with a shift to left. Her erythrocyte sedimentation rate was 96. Liver enzymes were significantly elevated, serum protein was low, and she was positive for hepatitis B. Her HIV test was negative. The neurosurgeon felt that the need for immediate decompression of Cam's spinal cord outweighed the information that a CT-myelogram could provide, so Cam was taken directly to the operating room for a decompressive laminectomy and drainage of her epidural abscess. Blood cultures taken in the emergency room were positive for methicillin-resistant staphylococcus. Pus drained from the abscess was gram positive and ultimately grew out methicillin-resistant staphylococcus. Cam began a long course of antibiotics and therapy. After 3.5 months on the rehabilitation unit, Cam was able to walk with the assistance of a walker. We cured the disease. . .but how were we going to cure the patient? Like I have said. . .some patients really break your heart.

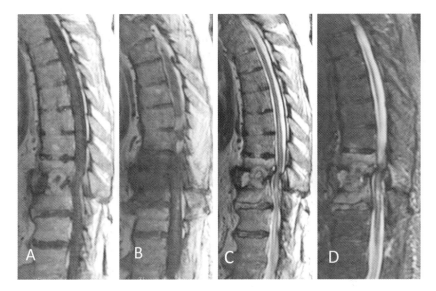

Fig. 8.3 Magnetic resonance imaging (MRI) images include a sagittal T1 with (A) and without (B) contrast, (C) T2, and (D) short tau inversion recovery (STIR). demonstrating osteomyelitis, infectious discitis, and an epidural abscess at the T9–T10 interspace. (From Masdeu J, Gilberto-Gonzalez R. *Handbook of Clinical Neurology*. Vol. 136. Amsterdam: Elsevier; 2016: Fig. 52.8.)

 Clinical Correlation—Putting It All Together

What is the diagnosis?
- T11 paraparesis secondary to spinal epidural abscess

The Science Behind the Diagnosis
EPIDURAL ABSCESS

Epidural abscess is an uncommon cause of spine pain that if undiagnosed, can result in paralysis and life-threatening complications. Epidural abscess can occur anywhere in the spine as well as intracranially (Fig. 8.4). It can occur spontaneously via hematogenous seeding, most frequently as a result of urinary tract infections that spread to the spinal epidural space via Batson's plexus. More commonly, epidural abscess occurs after intravenous drug use and instrumentation of the spine, including surgery and epidural nerve blocks (Box 8.1).

A patient with spinal epidural abscess initially presents with ill-defined pain in the segment of the spine affected (e.g., cervical, thoracic, or lumbar). This pain becomes more intense and localized as the abscess increases in size and compresses neural structures. Low-grade fever and vague constitutional symptoms, including malaise and anorexia, progress to frank sepsis with a high-grade fever,

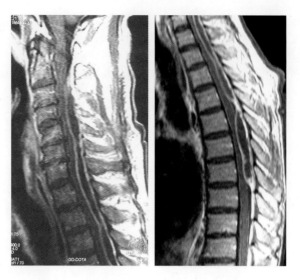

Fig. 8.4   Sagittal T_1-weighted magnetic resonance image (MRI) with gadolinium enhancement, revealing a posterior spinal epidural abscess from C2 to T8. (From Payer M, Walser H. Evacuation of a 14-vertebral-level cervico-thoracic epidural abscess and review of surgical options for extensive spinal epidural abscesses. *J Clin Neurosci.* 2008;15(4):483–486, Fig 1.)

BOX 8.1 ■ Causes of Epidural Abscess

- Spinal instrumentation
- Spinal injections
- Epidural catheters
- Epidural administration of steroids
- Intravenous drug abuse
- Contiguous bony infection
- Contiguous soft tissue infection
- Hematogenous spread from distant locations (e.g., dental abscess)
- Infectious endocarditis
- Tattooing
- Hemodialysis catheters

---

rigors, and chills. At this point, the patient begins to experience sensory and motor deficits and bowel and bladder symptoms as the result of neural compromise. As the abscess continues to expand, compromise of the vascular supply to the affected spinal cord and nerve occurs with resultant ischemia and if untreated, infarction and permanent neurologic deficits.

The patient with spinal epidural abscess often presents with the classic triad of fever, spinal pain, and neurologic deficits (Fig. 8.5). Initially, the epidural pain may be ill defined in the general area of the infection. The neurologic examination is initially within normal limits. A low-grade fever, night

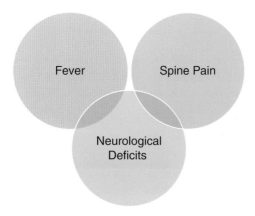

Fig. 8.5 The classic triad of spinal epidural abscess.

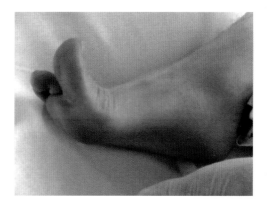

Fig. 8.6 Babinski sign. (From Ambesh P, Paliwal VK, Shetty V, Kamholz S. The Babinski sign: a comprehensive review. *J Neurol Sci.* 2017;372:477−481, Fig. 4.)

sweats, or both may be present. Theoretically, if the patient has received steroids or is immunocompromised, these constitutional symptoms may be attenuated or their onset may be delayed. As the abscess increases in size, the patient appears acutely ill, with fever, rigors, and chills. The clinician may be able to identify neurologic findings suggestive of spinal nerve root compression, spinal cord compression, or both. Subtle findings that point toward the development of myelopathy (e.g., Babinski's sign, clonus, and decreased perineal sensation) may be overlooked if not carefully sought (Fig. 8.6). As compression of the involved neural structures continues, the patient's neurologic status may deteriorate rapidly. If the diagnosis is not made, irreversible motor and sensory deficit occurs.

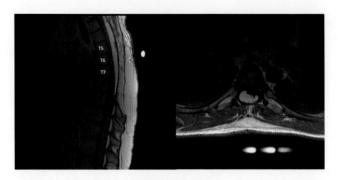

Fig. 8.7 *Left*: A recurrent spinal tumor extends from T2 to T9 with the spinal cord compression and tethered dorsally in contrast-enhanced T1-weighted magnetic resonance imaging (MRI); *Right*: Axial MRI at T5 level demonstrates severe spinal cord compression by tumor. (From Chen K-Y, Osorio J, Rivera J, Chou D. Intramedullary and extramedullary thoracic spinal lipomas without spinal dysraphism: clinical presentation and surgical management. *World Neurosurg.* 2019;121:156–159, Fig. 1.)

In this era of readily available magnetic resonance imaging (MRI) and high-speed computed tomography (CT), it may be more prudent to perform this noninvasive testing first rather than wait for a radiologist or spine surgeon to perform a myelogram. MRI and CT are highly accurate in the diagnosis of epidural abscess, with MRI becoming positive relatively early in the course of the disease. MRI also has the advantage of accurate diagnosis of intrinsic disease of the spinal cord and spinal tumor (Fig. 8.7). All patients suspected of having an epidural abscess should undergo laboratory testing consisting of complete blood cell count, erythrocyte sedimentation rate, C-reactive protein, and automated blood chemistries. Blood and urine cultures should be performed immediately in all patients thought to have epidural abscess to allow immediate implementation of antibiotic therapy while the workup is in progress. Gram stains and cultures of the abscess material also should be performed, but antibiotic treatment should not be delayed waiting for this information.

The diagnosis of epidural abscess should be strongly considered in any patient with spine pain and fever, especially if the patient has undergone spinal instrumentation or epidural nerve blocks for either surgical anesthesia or pain control or has a history of IV drug abuse. Other pathologic processes that must be considered in the differential diagnosis include intrinsic disease of the spinal cord, such as demyelinating disease and syringomyelia, and other pathology that can result in compression of the spinal cord and exiting nerve roots, such as metastatic tumor, Paget's disease, and neurofibromatosis (Fig. 8.8) (Box 8.2). As a general rule, unless the patient has concomitant infection, these diseases are routinely associated with only back pain and not with fever.

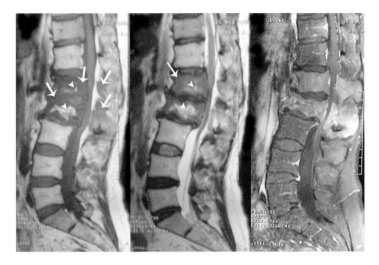

Fig. 8.8 Paget disease. Sagittal T1- (*left*) and T2-weighted (*middle*) magnetic resonance images of the lumbar spine revealed low signal intensity in the enlarged L1 and L2 vertebral bodies and posterior elements (*arrows*). There is preservation of the intraosseous fat, a useful discriminant from malignant infiltration (*arrowheads*). Postcontrast image (*right*) revealed enhancement of L1 and L2 vertebrae caused by increased blood supply. (From Demir MK, Yapıcıer Ö, Toktaş ZO. Lumbar Paget disease with spinal stenosis and conus medullaris compression. *Spine J.* 2016;16(1):e51—e52, Fig. 2.)

BOX 8.2 ■ Risk Factors for Spinal Epidural Abscess

- Spinal/epidural injections
- Epidural administration of steroids
- Epidural catheters
- Spinal instrumentation
- Diabetes mellitus
- Central lines
- Immunosuppression
- Alcoholism
- HIV infection
- Cirrhosis
- Malignancy
- Pregnancy
- Implantable devices

ANATOMY OF THE EPIDURAL SPACE

The superior boundary of the epidural space is the fusion of the periosteal and spinal layers of dura at the foramen magnum. The epidural space continues inferiorly to the sacrococcygeal membrane. The epidural space is bounded anteriorly

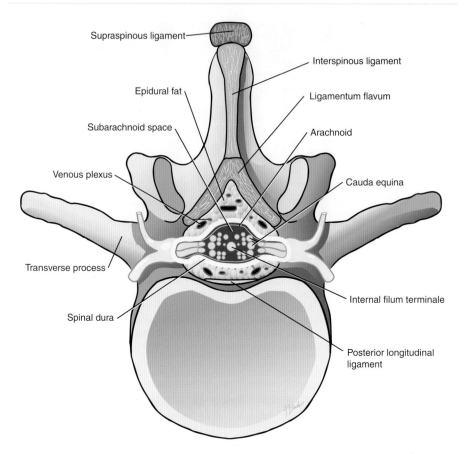

Fig. 8.9 Anatomy of the epidural space. (From Waldman SD, Bloch J. *Pain Management*. Philadelphia: Saunders; 2007:687, Fig. 20.7.)

by the posterior longitudinal ligament and posteriorly by the vertebral laminae and the ligamentum flavum (Fig. 8.9). The vertebral pedicles and intervertebral foramina form the lateral limits of the epidural space. The distance between the ligamentum flavum and dura is greatest at the L2 interspace, measuring 5 to 6 mm in the adult. Because of the enlargement of the cervical spinal cord corresponding to the neuromeres serving the upper extremities, this distance is decreased to 1.5 to 2.0 mm at the seventh cervical vertebra.

The epidural space is filled with fatty areolar tissue. The amount of epidural fat varies in direct proportion to the amount of fat stored elsewhere in the body. The epidural fat is relatively vascular and appears to change to a denser consistency with aging. This change in consistency may account for the significant variations in required drug dosage in adults, especially when utilizing the caudal approach to the epidural space. The epidural fat appears to perform two functions: (1) It serves as a shock absorber for the other contents of the epidural space

> **BOX 8.3 ■ Mechanisms of Spinal Cord Damage From Epidural Abscess**
>
> - Direct mechanical compression
> - Thrombosis of adjacent veins
> - Thrombophlebitis of adjacent veins
> - Disruption of spinal cord arterial supply
> - Local inflammatory response
> - Bacterial toxins

as well as the dura and the contents of the dural sac, and (2) It serves as a depot for drugs injected into the cervical epidural space. This second function has direct clinical implications when choosing opioids for cervical epidural administration.

The epidural veins are concentrated primarily in the anterolateral portion of the epidural space. These veins are valveless and hence transmit both the intrathoracic and intraabdominal pressures. As pressures in either of these body cavities increase owing to the Valsalva maneuver or to compression of the inferior vena cava by the gravid uterus or tumor mass, the epidural veins distend and decrease the volume of the epidural space. This decrease in volume can directly affect the volume of drug needed to obtain a given level of neural blockade. Because this venous plexus serves the entire spinal column, it acts as a ready conduit for the spread of hematogenous infection. The arteries that supply the bony and ligamentous confines of the epidural space as well as the spinal cord enter the cervical epidural space via two routes: (1) the intervertebral foramina and (2) direct anastomoses from the intracranial portions of the vertebral arteries. There are significant anastomoses between the epidural arteries. The epidural arteries lie primarily in the lateral portions of the epidural space. Trauma to the epidural arteries can result in epidural hematoma formation and/or compromise of the blood supply of the spinal cord itself. Compression of the epidural arteries by abscess or tumor can result in spinal cord ischemia and infarction (Box 8.3). The lymphatics of the epidural space are concentrated in the region of the dural roots, where they remove foreign material from the subarachnoid and epidural space.

MANAGEMENT AND TREATMENT

The rapid initiation of treatment of epidural abscess is mandatory if the patient is to avoid the sequelae of permanent neurologic deficit or death. The treatment of epidural abscess has two goals: (1) treatment of the infection with antibiotics and (2) drainage of the abscess to relieve compression on neural structures. Because most epidural abscesses are caused by *Staphylococcus aureus*, antibiotics such as vancomycin, which treat staphylococcal infection, should be started immediately after blood and urine culture samples are taken. Antibiotic therapy can be tailored to the culture and sensitivity reports as they become available. As mentioned, antibiotic therapy should not be delayed while waiting for a definitive diagnosis if epidural abscess is being considered as part of the differential diagnosis.

Antibiotics alone rarely treat an epidural abscess successfully unless the diagnosis is made very early in the course of the disease; drainage of the abscess is required to effect full recovery. Drainage of the epidural abscess is usually accomplished via decompression laminectomy and evacuation of the abscess. More recently, interventional radiologists have been successful in draining epidural abscesses percutaneously using drainage catheters placed with the use of CT or MRI guidance. Serial CT or MRI scans are useful in following the resolution of epidural abscess; scans should be repeated immediately at the first sign of a negative change in the patient's neurologic status. The clinician must always be cognizant of the fact that more than one pathologic process may be responsible for the patient's symptomatology and that compromise of the spinal cord may occur at more than one level.

HIGH-YIELD TAKEAWAYS

- The patient has the classic triad of symptoms associated with spinal epidural abscess.
- The patient's neurologic examination is grossly abnormal, with paraparesis suggestive of an incomplete spinal cord lesion.
- Pathologic reflexes are present and suggestive of myelopathy.
- There is decreased anal sphincter tone.
- There is decreased perineal sensation.
- The clinician should have a high index of suspicion of spinal epidural abscess in febrile IV drug abusers.
- MRI scanning is highly sensitive in the diagnosis of spinal epidural abscess.
- Paraparesis is a significant finding and may require urgent surgical intervention to avoid disastrous neurologic sequalae.

Suggested Readings

Akter F, Kotter M. Pathobiology of degenerative epidural abscess. *Neurosurg Clin North Am*. 2018;29(1):13—19.

Badhiwala JH, Wilson JR. The natural history of degenerative epidural abscess. *Neurosurg Clin North Am*. 2018;29(1):21—32.

Bhise V, Meyer AND, Singh H, et al. Errors in diagnosis of spinal epidural abscesses in the era of electronic health records. *Am J Med*. 2017;130(8):975−981.

Cetinkaya A, Pierre-Jerome C. Simultaneous occurrence of spinal epidural abscess and disk herniation causing irreversible neurologic deficits: a case report and review of the literature. *Radiology Case Reports*. 2018;13(3):719−723.

Prasad GL. Spinal epidural abscess—conservative or operative approach: a management dilemma. *World Neurosurgery*. 2017;103:945−947.

Shah AA, Yang H, Ogink PT, Schwab JH. Independent predictors of spinal epidural abscess recurrence. *The Spine Journal*. 2018:18(10):1837−1844.

Vakili M, Crum-Cianflone NF. Spinal epidural abscess: a series of 101 cases. *Am J Med*. 2017;130(12):1458−1463.

Dre Love

A 28-Year-Old Male With Acute Low Back Pain

- Learn the common causes of lumbar strain.
- Learn the clinical presentation of lumbar strain.
- Learn to distinguish lumbar strain from lumbar radiculopathy.
- Learn the anatomic structures affected by lumbar strain.
- Develop an understanding of the treatment options for lumbar strain.
- Develop an understanding of the role of physical therapy in the treatment of lumbar strain.
- Develop an understanding of the role in interventional pain management in the treatment of lumbar strain.

Dre Love

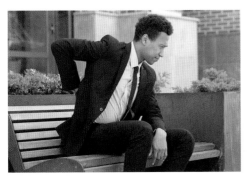

Dre Love is a 28-year-old paralegal with the chief complaint of "my back is killing me." I asked Dre when the pain began and he told me that it started about a week ago when he was lifting heavy boxes of files out of the trunk of his car. I asked him to show me where the pain was. He used the palm of his hand to rub the right side of his back. I then asked did the pain go into his legs and he said no . . . just the back . . . mostly on the right side and a little on the left. He denied any numbness, tingling, or weakness in his legs or feet, but noted that his back muscles "felt tight."

Dre described the pain as a "deep, dull ache" that worsened when he got up from his chair, got out of his car, or tried to stand up straight. He said that he felt "like an old man because when he bent over to the left and couldn't stand up straight." Dre went on to say that he was really tired from having to sleep in a chair at night. He went on to say that court could be pretty boring, and he was afraid that he would fall asleep in front of the judge. I asked him what he had been doing to manage the pain and he said he had tried over-the-counter Advil, a lidocaine patch, and a heating pad, but nothing really worked. He said he had tried Tylenol PM to help him sleep, but all it did was make him feel fuzzy and hung over.

On physical examination, Dre was afebrile and normotensive. His head, ears, eyes, nose, and throat (HEENT) examination, including a careful fundoscopic examination, was completely normal, as was his cardiopulmonary examination. A supernumerary nipple was noted on the left. His abdominal examination revealed a small umbilical hernia. There was no abnormal mass or organomegaly and no peripheral edema. Dre's neurologic examination was normal. Specifically, his upper and lower extremity deep tendon reflexes were physiologic and there was no sensory deficit or weakness.

Examination of the back revealed that Dre was sitting stiffly on the edge of the examination table, trying his best to splint his back. Palpation of the muscles of the lower back revealed tenderness to deep palpation bilaterally. There was moderate muscle spasm and muscle tightness greater on the right than on the left. There were no myofascial trigger points. Decreased active and passive flexion with a marked exacerbation of pain on extension of the lumbar spine was noted (Figs. 9.1 and 9.2). The Lasegue test was negative bilaterally. I asked Dre to get up and walk. He got up with great difficulty and I noted lateral shifting of the lumbar spine (a list to the right) and an antalgic gait as he walked down the

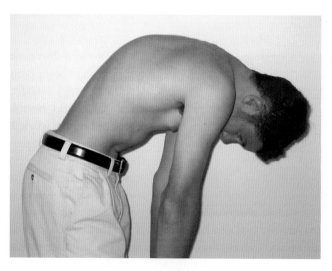

Fig. 9.1 Flexion of the lumbar spine. (From Waldman SD. *Physical Diagnosis of Pain: An Atlas of Signs and Symptoms*. 3rd ed. Philadelphia: Elsevier; 2016: Fig. 140.1.)

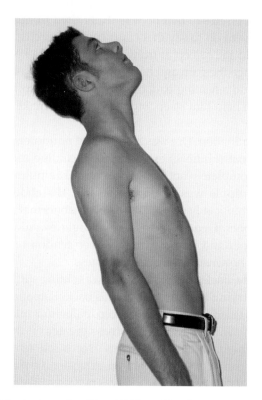

Fig. 9.2 Extension of the lumbar spine. (From Waldman SD. *Physical Diagnosis of Pain: An Atlas of Signs and Symptoms*. 3rd ed. Philadelphia: Elsevier; 2016: Fig. 140.2.)

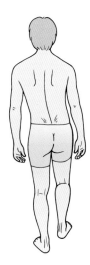

Fig. 9.3 Lateral shifting (lumbar list). (From Norris C. *Managing Sports Injuries*. 4th ed. Philadelphia; London: Churchill Livingstone; 2011: Fig. 13.9C.)

hall (Fig. 9.3). No pathologic reflexes or clonus were identified. Dre denied bowel and bladder symptoms associated with his pain.

Key Clinical Points—What's Important and What's Not

THE HISTORY

- Chief complaint of "my back is killing me"
- Significant sleep disturbance associated with pain
- Recent history of injuring back while lifting heavy boxes out of the trunk of his car
- Lack of significant antecedent trauma to back (e.g., motor vehicle accident, fall)
- Back stiffness and tightness
- Inability to stand up straight
- Feels like he is leaning to the right (see Fig. 9.3)
- No pain radiating into lower extremities
- No numbness or weakness of lower extremities
- Symptoms triggered by flexion and extension of the lumbar spine
- No urinary or fecal incontinence
- No pathologic reflexes

THE PHYSICAL EXAMINATION

- The patient is afebrile
- Back posturing in an attempt to splint back
- Lumbar lateral shifting (list) present (see Fig. 9.3)

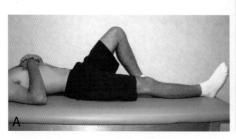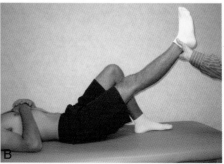

Fig. 9.4 Lasègue's straight leg raising test. (A) With the patient in the supine position, the unaffected leg is flexed 45 degrees at the knee and the affected leg is placed flat against the table. (B) With the ankle of the affected leg placed at 90 degrees of flexion, the affected leg is slowly raised toward the ceiling while the knee is kept fully extended. (From Waldman SD. *Atlas of Common Pain Syndromes*. 4th ed. Philadelphia: Elsevier; 2016: Fig. 82.2.)

- Normal deep tendon reflexes
- Normal upper and lower extremity motor and sensory examination
- No pathologic reflexes
- No clonus
- Negative Lasegue sign (Fig. 9.4)

OTHER FINDINGS OF NOTE

- Normal cardiovascular examination
- Normal pulmonary examination
- Normal abdominal examination
- No peripheral edema
- Umbilical hernia
- Supernumerary nipple

 What Tests Would You Like to Order?

The following tests were ordered:
- Lumbar spine radiographs.

Given his physical examination and the lack of significant antecedent trauma (e.g., motor vehicle accident, fall), I decided to wait on ordering an MRI of the lumbar spine. I made a note to have Dre see a general surgeon to take a look at his umbilical hernia.

TEST RESULTS

Dre's lumbar spine radiographs were normal. There was no bony abnormality (Fig. 9.5).

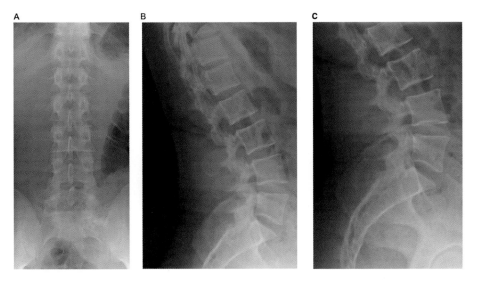

Fig. 9.5 Lumbar spine radiographs. (A) Standard AP view of the lumbar spine. Visualization from mid T11 to upper sacrum. (B) Standard lateral view of the lumbar spine. Visualization from T11 to upper sacrum. (C) Standard lumbosacral junction radiograph. *AP,* Anteroposterior. (From Jo AS, Wilseck Z, Manganaro MS, Ibrahim M. Essentials of spine trauma imaging: radiographs, CT, and MRI. *Semin Ultrasound CT MR.* 2018;39(6):532−550.)

📋 Clinical Correlation—Putting It All Together

What is the diagnosis?
- Lumbar strain

The Science Behind the Diagnosis
LUMBAR STRAIN

Acute lumbar strain is a constellation of symptoms consisting of nonradicular back pain that may radiate in a nondermatomal pattern into the low back and hips. Lumbar strain is usually the result of overuse injury, trauma, and stretch injury associated muscles and ligaments (Fig. 9.6). Lumbar strain can occur from acute injuries, such as motor vehicle accidents or lifting injuries, or it may simply develop over time as a result of repetitive stress or overuse injuries. Complicating the diagnosis, other causes of low back pain may be incorrectly attributed to seemingly minor low back injuries (Box 9.1). The clinician must always be alert to red flags in the history and physical examination that suggest that a more serious etiology may be responsible for a patient's low back pain (Box 9.2).

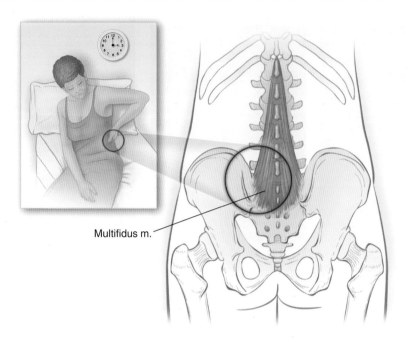

Multifidus m.

Fig. 9.6 Lumbar strain is usually the result of overuse injury, trauma, and stretch injury associated muscles and ligaments. (From Waldman SD. *Atlas of Uncommon Pain Syndromes*. 3rd ed. Philadelphia: Saunders; 2014: Fig. 81.1.)

BOX 9.1 ■ Differential Diagnosis of Low Back Pain

Mechanical Etiology
- Degenerative disc disease
- Facet arthropathy
- Spinal stenosis
- Spondylolisthesis
- Spondylolysis
- Traumatic transverse process fracture
- Kyphosis
- Scoliosis
- Congenital abnormalities of the vertebra (e.g., transitional vertebra, trefoil canal)

Nonmechanical Etiology
- Primary neoplasm
- Metastatic disease
- Osteomyelitis
- Multiple myeloma
- Paget disease of bone

(Continued)

- Myofascial pain
- Discitis
- Epidural abscess
- Paraspinal abscess
- Retroperitoneal tumors
- Spinal cord tumors
- Lymphoma
- Leukemia
- Herpes zoster
- Anklylosing spondylitis
- Reiter syndrome
- Psoriatic arthritis
- Scheuermann's disease
- Visceral disease
- Pancreatitis
- Renal calculi
- Ureteral calculi
- Cholecystitis
- Posterior penetrating gastric ulcer
- Idiopathic

BOX 9.2 ■ Red Flags in Patients Suffering From Low Back Pain

- History of significant trauma
- Nonmechanical back pain
- Past history of cancer
- Unexplained fever
- Unexplained weight loss or inanition
- Bony abnormality
- Abnormal neurologic examination
- Altered sensorium
- Presence of pathologic reflexes
- Alterations of gait

THE MUSCLES OF THE BACK

The muscles of the back work together as a functional unit to stabilize and allow both coordinated movement of the low back and maintenance of an upright position. Trauma to an individual muscle can result in dysfunction of the entire functional unit. The rhomboids, latissimus dorsi, iliocostalis quadratus lumborum, multifidus, and psoas muscles are subject to lumbar strain The points of origin and attachments of these muscles are particularly susceptible to trauma and the subsequent development of myofascial trigger points (Fig. 9.7). Injection of these trigger points serves as a diagnostic and therapeutic maneuver. Spondylosis, degenerative facet joint arthritis, and degenerative disc disease may contribute to the symptoms associated with lumbar strain.

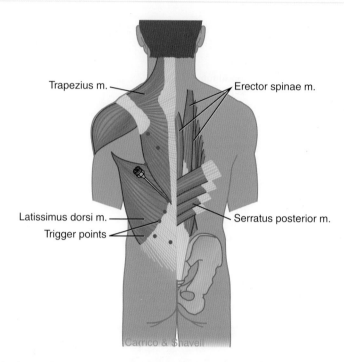

Fig. 9.7 Injection technique to relieve lumbar myofascial pain. (From Waldman SD. *Atlas of Uncommon Pain Syndromes*. 3rd ed. Philadelphia: Saunders; 2014: Fig. 81.2.)

MANAGEMENT AND TREATMENT

Lumbar strain is best treated with a multimodality approach (Box 9.3). Physical therapy, including heat modalities and deep sedative massage, combined with simple analgesics, nonsteroidal anti inflammatory drugs, and skeletal muscle relaxants, is a reasonable starting point. Identification and correction of abnormal ergonomic factors contributing to repetitive stress and overuse injuries is key to successful treatment of lumbar strain. If myofascial trigger points are identified, trigger point injections may be useful. The use of botulinum toxin A trigger point injections may offer symptomatic relief in selected patients. Gentle manipulative therapy and soft tissue techniques are useful adjuncts in the management of lumbar strain. Some patients will experience relief with the use of acupuncture and transcutaneous nerve stimulation. Opioid analgesics should be avoided in this patient population, because the risks outweigh the benefits.

In patients who do not respond to conservative treatment, lumbar epidural block, blockade of the medial branch of the dorsal ramus, or intraarticular injection of the facet joint with local anesthetic and steroids is extremely effective and may be a reasonable next step (Fig. 9.8). Underlying sleep disturbance and depression are best treated with a tricyclic antidepressant such as nortriptyline,

BOX 9.3 ■ Treatment Modalities for Lumbar Strain

Physical Modalities
- Physical therapy
- Local heat
- Deep sedative massage
- Ice rubs

Medication Management
- Simple analgesics
- Nonsteroidal anti inflammatory agents
- Skeletal muscle relaxants

Acupuncture
TENS Unit
  Manipulative Therapy
  Interventional Pain Management
- Trigger point injections
- Medial branch block
- Lumbar epidural block
  TENS, Transcutaneous electrical nerve stimulator

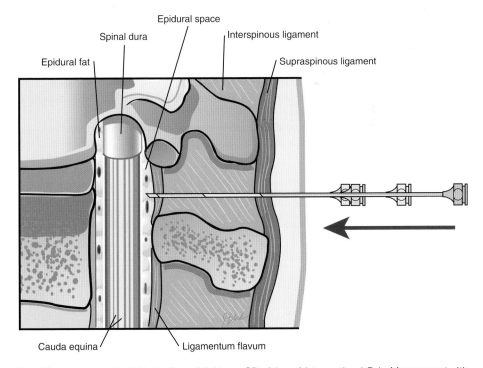

Fig. 9.8 Lumbar epidural block. (From Waldman SD. *Atlas of Interventional Pain Management.* 4th ed. Philadelphia: Saunders; 2015: Fig. 97.8.)

which can be started at a single bedtime dose of 25 mg. The tricyclic antidepressants should be used with care in the elderly.

HIGH-YIELD TAKEAWAYS

- The patient's symptomatology is the result of a lifting injury rather than more severe acute trauma, making bony abnormality unlikely.
- The patient's pain is localized in the lower back without radiation into the lower extremities, which makes the diagnosis of lumbar radiculopathy less likely.
- The patient is afebrile, making an infectious etiology unlikely.
- The patient's neurologic examination is normal; specifically, there is no sensory deficit or muscle weakness and deep tendon reflexes are normal, making a diagnosis of lumbar radiculopathy unlikely.
- There are no bowel or bladder symptoms or pathologic reflexes suggestive of myelopathy.
- The patient has significant sleep disturbance.
- Many pathologic processes can present as low back pain (see Box 9.1).

Suggested Reading

Hartvigsen J, Hancock MJ, Kongsted A, et al. What low back pain is and why we need to pay attention. *Lancet.* 2018;391(10137):2356–2367.

Maher C, Underwood M, Buchbinder R. Non-specific low back pain. *Lancet.* 2017;389 (10070):736–747.

Qaseem A, Wilt TJ, McLean RM, Forciea MA. Noninvasive treatments for acute, sub-acute, and chronic low back pain: a clinical practice guideline from the American College of Physicians. *Ann Intern Med.* 2017;166(7):514–530.

Tan A, Zhou J, Kuo YF, Goodwin JSD. Variation among primary care physicians in the use of imaging for older patients with acute low back pain. *J Gen Intern Med.* 2016;31:156–163.

Andy "Axel" Rhodes

A 42-Year-Old Male With Acute Low Back Pain That Radiates Into His Shin With Associated Numbness

- Learn the common causes of lumbar radiculopathy.
- Develop an understanding of the role of the intervertebral disc in lumbar radiculopathy.
- Learn the clinical presentation of lumbar radiculopathy.
- Learn how to use physical examination to determine which lumbar spinal nerve roots are subserving the patient's pain.
- Learn to distinguish lumbar strain from lumbar radiculopathy.
- Learn the important anatomic structures in lumbar radiculopathy.
- Develop an understanding of the treatment options for lumbar radiculopathy.
- Learn the appropriate testing options to help diagnose lumbar radiculopathy.
- Learn to identify red flags waving in patients who present with lumbar radiculopathy.
- Develop an understanding of the role of interventional pain management in the treatment of lumbar radiculopathy.

Andy "Axel" Rhodes

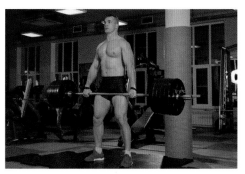

Andy "Axel" Rhodes is a 42-year-old bartender with a chief complaint of, "My back is really screwed up." Axel went on to say, "While power lifting over at Gold's Gym a few weeks ago, all of a sudden, one of the weights shifted and when I tried to catch it, I wrenched my back." I asked, "So, Axel, have you ever had anything like this before?" He said, "Not really. A couple of times, I've bunged up my back when I was working as a bouncer and had to get up close and personal with someone who getting out of line . . . but no . . . never anything that hurts like this and never anything with pain going into my legs."

"Axel, I want you to point with one finger to show me where it hurts the most." He pointed to the right side of his lower lumbar spine. "It really hurts all around here and shoots down into my thigh and goes down all the way to my right shin. A lot of times, it feels like my leg has gone to sleep. The leg just doesn't feel right. It's getting really hard to use the kick starter to start my bike."

On physical examination, Axel was afebrile and normotensive. I started to look in Axel's eyes and he said, "Hey doctor, did you know there is a new website for people who suffer from chronic eye pain?' Before I could respond, he went on to say . . . "Yeah . . . it's a site for sore eyes." Try as I might, I couldn't keep from laughing as I went on with the physical examination. His head, ears, eyes, nose, and throat (HEENT) examination was normal, as was his cardiopulmonary examination. His abdominal examination revealed no abnormal mass or organomegaly. There was no peripheral edema. I noted that Axel was holding his back stiffly so as not to move it. Palpation of the lumbar paraspinous muscles revealed tenderness to deep palpation and pretty significant spasm of the paraspinous muscles, the right greater than the left. Axel grimaced when I stood him up and asked him to flex and extend his back. A careful neurologic examination of the lower extremities revealed a normal sensory examination on the left, but decreased sensation over the shin on the right (Fig. 10.1). He was moderately weak in the ankle dorsiflexors on the right (Fig. 10.2). The knee jerk reflex was normal on the left, but definitely diminished on the right (Fig. 10.3). His ankle jerks were physiologic bilaterally. Axel's upper extremity motor and sensory examination, as well as his upper extremity deep tendon reflexes, were normal. The Lasegue test was positive bilaterally (Fig. 10.4) No pathologic reflexes or clonus were identified. Axel denied bowel and bladder symptoms associated with his pain.

SENSORY

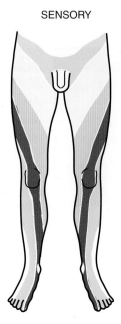

Fig. 10.1   Sensory distribution of the L4 dermatome (*purple*). (From Waldman SD. *Physical Diagnosis of Pain: An Atlas of Signs and Symptoms*. 3rd ed. St. Louis: Elsevier; 2016: Fig. 144.1.)

MOTOR

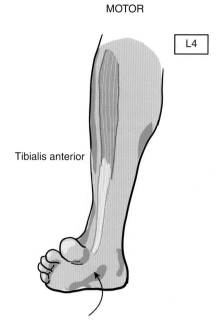

Fig. 10.2   L4 manual muscle testing. (From Waldman SD. *Physical Diagnosis of Pain: An Atlas of Signs and Symptoms*. 3rd ed. St. Louis: Elsevier; 2016: Fig. 144.2.)

REFLEX

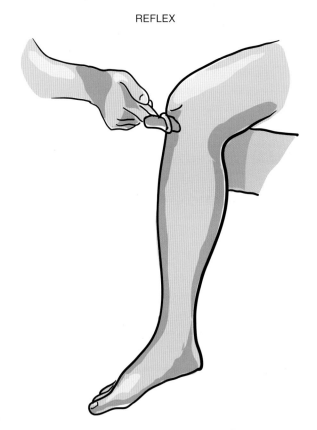

Fig. 10.3 Knee jerk (patellar) deep tendon reflex. (From Waldman SD. *Physical Diagnosis of Pain: An Atlas of Signs and Symptoms*. 3rd ed. St. Louis: Elsevier; 2016: Fig. 144.3.)

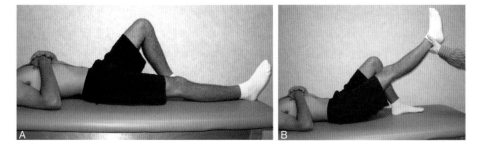

Fig. 10.4 (A) The Lasegue straight leg raising test. The patient is in the supine position with the unaffected leg flexed to 45 degrees at the knee and the affected leg placed flat against the table. (B) The Lasegue straight leg raising test. With the ankle of the affected leg placed at 90 degrees of flexion, the affected leg is slowly raised toward the ceiling while the knee is kept fully extended. (From Waldman SD. *Physical Diagnosis of Pain: An Atlas of Signs and Symptoms*. 3rd ed. St. Louis: Elsevier; 2016: Figs. 147.1 and 147.2.)

Key Clinical Points—What's Important and What's Not

THE HISTORY

- History of acute trauma—a weightlifting injury
- No significant history of previous back pain
- Back pain radiating from the low back into the right lower extremity
- Sensation that right leg "had gone to sleep"
- Difficulty using right leg to start his motorcycle
- No bowel or bladder symptomatology

THE PHYSICAL EXAMINATION

- The patient is afebrile
- Back posturing in an attempt to splint his back
- Diminished knee jerk reflex on right (see Fig. 10.3)
- Decreased sensation over the right shin (see Fig. 10.1)
- Weakness of the ankle dorsiflexors on the right (see Fig. 10.2)
- Normal left upper and lower extremity motor and sensory examination
- No pathologic reflexes
- No clonus
- Positive Lasegue sign bilaterally (see Fig. 10.4)

OTHER FINDINGS OF NOTE

- Normal HEENT examination
- Normal cardiovascular examination
- Normal pulmonary examination
- Normal abdominal examination
- No peripheral edema

 What Tests Would You Like to Order?

The following tests were ordered:
- MRI scan of the lumbar spine
- Electromyogram and nerve conduction studies of the left lower extremity

TEST RESULTS

The MRI scan of Axel's lumbar spine revealed a large right-sided lateral disc herniation at L4 (Fig. 10.5). The electromyogram was positive for acute denervation of the L4 innervated muscles on the right. Nerve conduction velocity test revealed no evidence of entrapment or peripheral neuropathy.

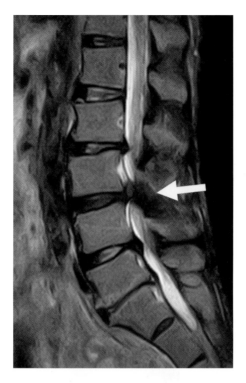

Fig. 10.5   Sagittal view of T1-weighted magnetic resonance image. Lumbar disk protrusion and compression of the spinal cord were most obvious at the L3-L4 level (*arrow*). (From Sawai T, Nakahira J, Minami T. Paraplegia caused by giant intradural herniation of a lumbar disk after combined spinal-epidural anesthesia in total hip arthroplasty. *J Clin Anesth*. 2016;32:169–171, Fig. 1.)

 # Clinical Correlation—Putting It All Together

What is the diagnosis?
- L4 radiculopathy on right

The Science Behind the Diagnosis

THE DERMATOMES AND MYOTOMES

In humans, the innervation of the skin, muscles, and deep structures is determined embryologically at an early stage of fetal development, and there is amazingly little intersubject variability. Each segment of the spinal cord and its corresponding spinal nerves have a consistent segmental relationship that allows the clinician to ascertain the probable spinal level of dysfunction based on the pattern of pain, muscle weakness, and deep tendon reflex changes.

In general, in humans, the more proximal the muscle, the more cephalad the spinal segment, with the ventral muscles innervated by higher spinal segments than the corresponding dorsal muscles (Figs. 10.6 and 10.7). Pain perceived in the region of a given muscle or joint may not be coming from that muscle or joint, but simply be referred by problems at the same lumbar spinal segment that innervates the muscles. Furthermore, the clinician needs to be aware that the relatively consistent pattern of dermatomal and myotomal distribution breaks down when the pain is perceived in the deep structures of the upper extremity (e.g., the joints and tendinous insertions). With pain in these regions, the clinician should refer to a sclerotomal chart.

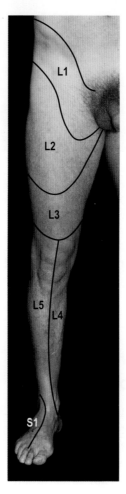

Fig. 10.6 Dermatomes of the lower extremity—anterior view. (From Jacob S. *Human Anatomy*. Philadelphia: Churchill Livingstone; 2008: Fig. 6.92.)

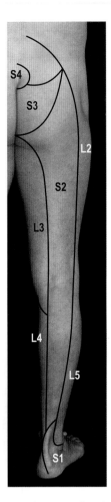

Fig. 10.7 Dermatomes of the lower extremity—posterior view. (From Jacob S. *Human Anatomy.* Philadelphia: Churchill Livingstone; 2008: Fig. 6.93.)

The concept of diagnosing a problem at a specific neurologic level via physical examination has its basis in the fact that pathology at the lumbar spinal cord or lumbar nerve root level manifests itself in a relatively consistent manner by dysfunction, numbness, and pain of the upper extremity, which occurs in a dermatomal distribution. Although not foolproof, a careful physical examination of the upper extremity with an eye to the neurologic level affected can frequently guide the clinician in designing a more targeted workup and treatment plan. By overlapping the information gleaned from physical examination with the neuroanatomic information gained from MRI and the neurophysiologic information from electromyography, a highly accurate diagnosis can be made as to what level of the lumbar spine is responsible for the patient's symptoms.

TABLE 10.1 ■ Clinical Features of Lumbar Radiculopathy

Lumbar Root	Pain	Sensory Changes	Weakness	Reflex Changes
L4 root	**Back, shin, thigh, leg**	**Shin numbness**	**Ankle dorsiflexors**	**Knee jerk**
L5 root	Back, posterior thigh, leg	Numbness, top of foot and first web space	Extensor hallucis longus	None
S1 root	Back, posterior calf, leg	Numbness, lateral foot	Gastrocnemius and soleus	Ankle jerk

Testing for the L4 dermatome is best carried out by a careful sensory evaluation of the skin overlying the shin on the affected lower extremity (see Fig. 10.1). Decreased sensation in this anatomic region can be ascribed to proximal lesions of the spinal cord, such as a spinal cord tumor or multiple sclerosis; to more distal lesions of the L4 nerve root, such as impingement by a herniated disc; or to a lesion of the more peripheral axillary nerve (see Fig. 10.5). For this reason, correlation with manual muscle testing and evaluation of the deep tendon reflex combined with radiographic and electromyographic testing can help to determine the exact site of pathology (Table 10.1).

Testing for the L4 myotome is best carried out by manual muscle testing of the ankle dorsiflexors. They are primarily innervated by the L4 spinal nerve. Because in most patients, dorsiflexion of the ankle is an L4 function, the muscles should be tested as follows. The patient is placed in the sitting position on the examination table. The patient is asked to dorsiflex the ankle against resistance (see Fig. 10.2). If the manual muscle testing is normal, the examiner should not be able to resist dorsiflexion.

The knee jerk deep tendon reflex is mediated via the L4 spinal segment. To test the knee jerk reflex, the patient is placed in the sitting position on the examination table and asked to relax. The clinician then strikes the patellar tendon with a neurologic hammer and grades the response (see Fig. 10.3). A diminished or absent reflex might point to compromise of the L4 segment, whereas a hyperactive response might suggest an upper motor neuron lesion, such as myelopathy.

LUMBAR RADICULOPATHY

Lumbar radiculopathy is a constellation of symptoms consisting of neurogenic back and lower extremity pain emanating from the lumbar nerve roots. In addition to the pain, the patient with lumbar radiculopathy may experience associated numbness, weakness, and loss of reflexes. The causes of lumbar radiculopathy include herniated disc, foraminal stenosis, tumor, osteophyte formation, and rarely, infection (Box 10.1). Many patients and their physicians will

> **BOX 10.1 ■ Causes of Lumbar Radiculopathy**
>
> - Herniated disc
> - Foraminal stenosis
> - Tumor
> - Osteophyte formation
> - Infection (rare)

use the term *sciatica* to refer to the constellation of symptoms known as lumbar radiculopathy.

SIGNS AND SYMPTOMS

The patient suffering from lumbar radiculopathy will complain of pain, numbness, tingling, and paresthesias in the distribution of the affected nerve root or roots (see Table 10.1). Patients may also note weakness and lack of coordination in the affected extremity. Muscle spasms and back pain, as well as pain referred into the buttocks, are common. Decreased sensation, weakness, and reflex changes are demonstrated on physical examination. Patients with lumbar radiculopathy will commonly experience a reflex shifting of the trunk to one side. This reflex shifting is called a lateral shift or a list. Occasionally, a patient suffering from lumbar radiculopathy will experience compression of the lumbar spinal nerve roots and cauda equina, resulting in myelopathy or cauda equina syndrome. Lumbar myelopathy is most commonly caused by a midline herniated lumbar disc, spinal stenosis, tumor, or rarely, infection. Patients suffering from lumbar myelopathy or cauda equina syndrome will experience varying degrees of lower extremity weakness and bowel and bladder symptomatology. This represents a neurosurgical emergency and should be treated as such.

TESTING

Magnetic resonance imaging of the lumbar spine will provide the clinician with the best information regarding the lumbar spine and its contents. MRI is highly accurate and will help identify abnormalities that may put the patient at risk for the development of lumbar myelopathy (Fig. 10.8). In patients who cannot undergo MRI (e.g., patients with a pacemaker), computed tomography or myelography is a reasonable second choice (Fig. 10.9). Discography may provide additional useful information in selected cases. Radionuclide bone scanning and plain radiographs are indicated if fracture or a bony abnormality, such as metastatic disease, is being considered. Although this testing provides the clinician with useful neuroanatomic information, electromyography and nerve conduction velocity testing will provide the clinician with neurophysiologic information

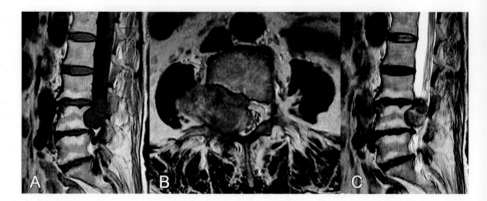

Fig. 10.8   T1-weighted sagittal MRI (A) and T2-weighted axial MRI (B) revealed a dumbbell lesion at L4/5 right intervertebral foramen. In the spinal canal, the upper part of the lesion is hypointense on T2-weighted sagittal image (C). (From Han Y, Lai X, Chen X, et al. Dumbbell schwannoma complicated by intradural lumbar disc herniation at the same level—a rare case report. *Interdiscipl Neurosurg.* 2019;18:1–3, Fig. 1.)

that can delineate the actual status of each individual nerve root and the lumbar plexus. Screening laboratory testing consisting of complete blood count, erythrocyte sedimentation rate, and automated blood chemistry testing should be performed if the diagnosis of lumbar radiculopathy is in question.

DIFFERENTIAL DIAGNOSIS

Lumbar radiculopathy is a clinical diagnosis that is supported by a combination of clinical history, physical examination, radiography, and MRI. Pain syndromes that may mimic lumbar radiculopathy include low back strain, lumbar bursitis, lumbar fibromyositis, inflammatory arthritis, and disorders of the lumbar spinal cord, roots, plexus, and nerves (Table 10.2). MRI of the lumbar spine should be carried out on all patients suspected of suffering from lumbar radiculopathy. Screening laboratory testing consisting of complete blood count, erythrocyte sedimentation rate, antinuclear antibody testing, HLA-B27 antigen screening, and automated blood chemistry testing should be performed if the diagnosis of lumbar radiculopathy is in question to help rule out other causes of the patient's pain.

THE INTERVERTEBRAL DISC

The lumbar intervertebral disc has two major functions. The first is to serve as the major shock-absorbing structure of the lumbar spine and the second is to facilitate the synchronized movement of the lumbar spine while helping to prevent impingement of the neural structures and vasculature that traverse the lumbar spine. Both the shock-absorbing function and the movement/protective function of the lumbar intervertebral disc are functions of the disc structure, as well as of the laws of physics that affect it.

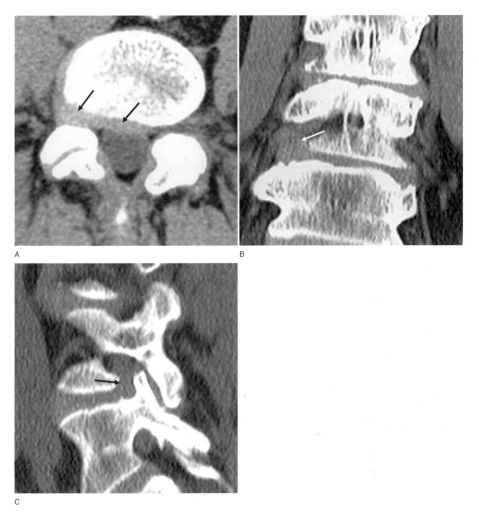

Fig. 10.9   Disc herniation. An acute disc herniation (*arrows*) is demonstrated on axial (A), coronal (B), and sagittal (C) multiplanar reconstructions. (From Waldman SD, Bloch J. *Pain Management*. Philadelphia: Saunders; 2007: Fig. 9.7.)

To understand how the lumbar intervertebral disc functions in health and becomes dysfunctional in disease, it is useful to think of the disc as a closed, fluid-filled container. The outside of the container is made up of a top and bottom, called the endplates, which are composed of relatively inflexible hyaline cartilage. The sides of the lumbar intervertebral disc are made up of a woven crisscrossing matrix of fibroelastic fibers that tightly attaches to the top and bottom endplates. This woven matrix of fibers is called the annulus, and it completely surrounds the sides of the disc (Fig. 10.10). The interlaced structure of the annulus results in an enclosing mesh that is extremely strong yet at the

TABLE 10.2 ■ **Clinical Syndromes That Can Mimic Low Back Pain and Lumbar Radiculopathy**

Localized Bony, Disc Space, or Joint Space Pathology	Primary Hip Pathology	Systemic Disease	Sympathetically Mediated Pain	Pain Referred from Other Body Areas
Vertebral fracture	Bursitis	Rheumatoid	Causalgia	Pancreatitis
Primary bone tumor	Tendinitis	arthritis	Reflex sympathetic	Malignancy of the
Facet joint disease	Aseptic	Collagen vascular	dystrophy	retroperitoneal
Localized or gener-	necrosis	disease	Postthrombophlebitis	space
alized degenerative	Osteoarthritis	Reiter syndrome	pain (milk leg)	Lumbar
arthritis	Joint instability	Gout		plexopathy
Osteophyte	Muscle strain	Other crystal		Fibromyalgia
formation	Muscle sprain	arthropathies		Myofascial pain
Disc space	Periarticular	Charcot neuro-		syndromes
infection	infection	pathic arthritis		Entrapment
Herniated lumbar	not involv-	Multiple sclerosis		neuropathies
disc	ing joint	Ischemic pain		Intraabdominal
Degenerative disc	space	secondary to		tumors
disease		peripheral		
Primary spinal cord		vascular		
and/or cauda		insufficiency		
equina		Ankylosing		
pathology		spondylitis		
Osteomyelitis				
Epidural abscess				
Epidural hematoma				

From Waldman SD. *Physical Diagnosis of Pain: An Atlas of Signs and Symptoms*. 3rd ed. St. Louis: Elsevier; 2016: Table 137.1.

same time very flexible, which facilitates the compression of the disc during the wide range of motion of the lumbar spine (Fig. 10.11).

Inside of this container consisting of the top and bottom endplates and surrounding annulus is the water-containing mucopolysaccharide gel-like substance called the nucleus pulposus (Fig. 10.12A). The nucleus is incompressible and transmits any pressure placed on one portion of the disc to the surrounding nucleus. In health, the water-filled gel creates a positive intradiscal pressure, which forces apart the adjacent vertebra and helps protect the spinal cord and exiting nerve roots. When the lumbar spine moves, the incompressible nature of the nucleus pulposus maintains a constant intradiscal pressure while some fibers of the disc relax and others contract.

As the lumbar intervertebral disc ages, it becomes less vascular and loses its ability to absorb water into the disc (Fig. 10.10B–D). This results in degradation of the disc's shock-absorbing and motion-facilitating functions. This problem worsens with degeneration of the annulus, which allows portions of the disc wall to bulge, distorting the ability of the nucleus pulposus to distribute evenly the forces placed on it throughout the entire disc. This exacerbates disc dysfunction and can contribute to further disc deterioration, which may ultimately lead

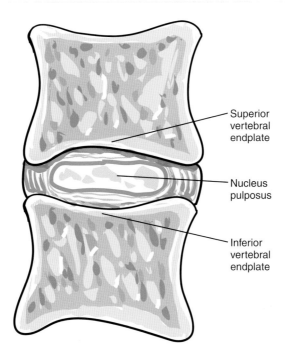

Fig. 10.10   Movement of adjacent lumbar vertebrae is allowed by three joints. The first comprises the inferior and superior endplates of the vertebral bodies and their interposed intervertebral disc. (From Waldman SD. *Physical Diagnosis of Pain: An Atlas of Signs and Symptoms*. 3rd ed. St. Louis: Elsevier; 2016: Fig. 135.2.)

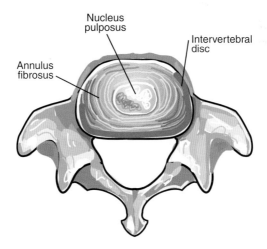

Fig. 10.11   The interlaced structure of the annulus results in an enclosing mesh that is extremely strong yet at the same time, very flexible, which facilitates the compression of the disc during the wide range of motion of the lumbar spine. (From Waldman SD. *Physical Diagnosis of Pain: An Atlas of Signs and Symptoms*. 3rd ed. St. Louis: Elsevier; 2016: Fig. 136.1.)

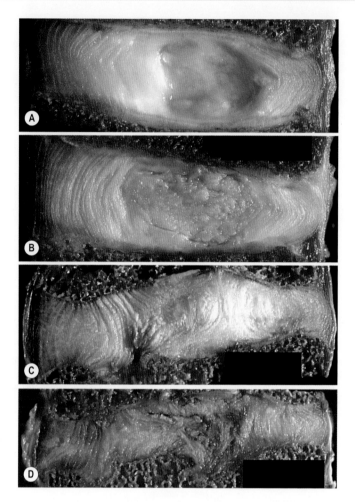

Fig. 10.12   Discal degeneration. (A) Healthy disc. (B) Early shrinkage. (C) Disc thinning with Schmorl's node formation. (D) Gross discal thinning and loss of disc height. (From Norris C. *Managing Sports Injuries*. 4th ed. Philadelphia: Churchill Livingstone; 2011: Fig. 13.5.)

to actual complete disruption of the annulus and extrusion of the nucleus. Intervertebral discs may herniate laterally, posteriorly, or anteriorly, as well as superiorly or inferiorly through weakened vertebral endplates (Fig. 10.13). The deterioration of the disc is responsible for many of the painful conditions emanating from the lumbar spine that are encountered in clinical practice.

MANAGEMENT AND TREATMENT

Lumbar radiculopathy is best treated with a multimodality approach. Physical therapy, including heat modalities and deep sedative massage, combined with

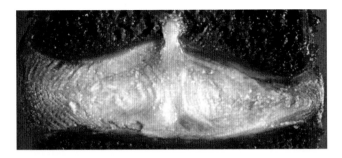

Fig. 10.13   Schmorl's node is indicative of vertebral endplate weakness. Note the herniation of nuclear material through the disc endplate. (Courtesy Steven Waldman, MD.)

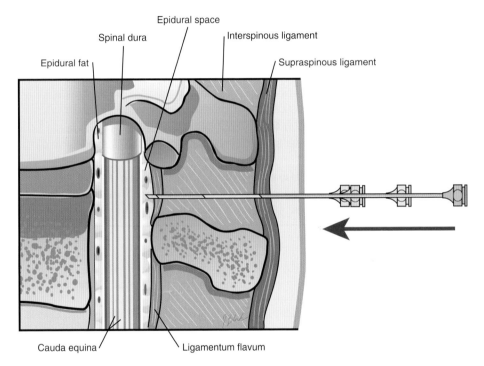

Fig. 10.14   With the operator applying constant pressure to the plunger of the syringe with the thumb of the right hand, the needle and syringe are continuously advanced in a slow and deliberate manner with the left hand. As soon as the needle bevel passes through the ligamentum flavum and enters the epidural space, there will be a sudden loss of resistance to injection, and the plunger will effortlessly surge forward. (From Waldman SD. *Atlas of Interventional Pain Management*. 4th ed. Philadelphia: Saunders; 2015: Fig. 97.8.)

nonsteroidal anti inflammatory agents and skeletal muscle relaxants, represents a reasonable starting point. The addition of lumbar steroid epidural nerve blocks is a reasonable next step (Fig. 10.14). Caudal or lumbar epidural blocks with local anesthetic and steroid have been shown to be extremely effective in the treatment of lumbar radiculopathy. Underlying sleep disturbance and depression are best treated with a tricyclic antidepressant compound, such as nortriptyline, which can be started at a single bedtime dose of 25 mg.

HIGH-YIELD TAKEAWAYS

- The patient is afebrile, making an acute infectious etiology (e.g., epidural abscess) unlikely.
- The patient's symptomatology is the result of acute trauma to the lumbar intervertebral disc.
- The patient's pain is localized in the back and right lower extremity, which is highly suggestive of lumbar radiculopathy.
- The patient's symptoms are unilateral, which would be more suggestive of lumbar radiculopathy vs. other pathologic processes, although bilateral radiculopathy is not that uncommon.
- The patient's neurologic examination is abnormal in the affected right lower extremity with L4 sensory deficit, ankle dorsiflexor weakness, and a diminished knee jerk reflex, which is highly suggestive of a right L4 radiculopathy.
- There are no bowel or bladder symptoms or pathologic reflexes suggestive of myelopathy.
- MRI scanning is highly sensitive in the diagnosis of discogenic disease and is useful in ruling out other space-occupying lesions that may be producing radicular symptoms (see Figs. 10.5 and 10.9).

Suggested Readings

Waldman SD. Functional anatomy of the lumbar spine. In: *Physical Diagnosis of Pain: An Atlas of Signs and Symptoms*. 4th ed. Philadelphia: Elsevier; 2020.

Waldman SD. Lumbar radiculopathy. In: *Pain Review*. 2nd ed. Philadelphia: Elsevier; 2017:256−257.

Barr K. Electrodiagnosis of lumbar radiculopathy. *Phys Med Rehabil Clin North Am.* 2013;24(1):79−91.

Waldman SD. Lumbar epidural nerve block: Interlaminar approach. In: *Atlas of Interventional Pain Management*. 4th ed. Philadelphia: Elsevier; 2015:500−513.

Waldman SD. The Lesegue straight leg raising test for lumbar radiculopathy. In: *Physical Diagnosis of Pain: An Atlas of Signs and Symptoms*. 3rd ed. Philadelphia: Elsevier; 2016:235−236.

Waldman SD, Campbell RSD. Anatomy: special imaging considerations of the lumbar spine. In: *Imaging of Pain*. Philadelphia: Elsevier; 2011:109−110.

Doris Chopp

A 58-Year-Old Female With Right Leg Weakness and Back Pain

- Learn the common causes of lumbar radiculopathy.
- Develop an understanding of the role of the intervertebral disc in lumbar radiculopathy.
- Develop an understanding of the causes of lumbar radiculopathy.
- Develop an understanding of the aging lumbar spine.
- Learn the clinical presentation of lumbar radiculopathy.
- Learn how to use physical examination to determine which lumbar spinal nerve roots are subserving the patient's pain.
- Learn to distinguish lumbar strain from lumbar radiculopathy.
- Learn the important anatomic structures in lumbar radiculopathy.
- Develop an understanding of the treatment options for lumbar radiculopathy.
- Learn the appropriate testing options to help diagnose lumbar radiculopathy.
- Learn to identify red flags waving in patients who present with lumbar radiculopathy.
- Develop an understanding of the role in interventional pain management in the treatment of lumbar radiculopathy.

Doris Chopp

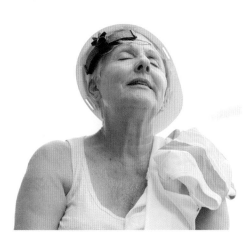

Doris Chopp is a 58-year-old construction worker with the chief complaint of "my right leg kept giving out." Doris went on to say that she wouldn't have bothered coming in, but she couldn't climb up onto the roof to see what her roofers were up to. I asked Doris if she had had anything like this happen before. She shook her head and responded, "just the usual aches and pains... you can't work construction and not have your back go out now and then...usually I just take a handful of aspirin and get right back on the horse. What worries me this time is the leg. I spend all day long climbing in and out of heavy equipment, up and down ladders, climbing over construction debris... I need to be able to rely on my legs...it is simply too dangerous otherwise."

I asked Doris to point with one finger to show me where it hurts the most. She pointed to the right side of her lower lumbar spine. "Look doctor, I can live with the back pain...it hurts all across my low back...but it's the right leg that is really the problem. I never know when it is going to give out. Sometimes, for no reason, I get an electric shock down the back of my right leg and the leg feels like it wants to buckle." "Is there any numbness?" I asked. "Yes. It is numb across the top of my foot and sometimes on the back of my leg." "Are you having any problem peeing or pooping?" I asked. "Absolutely not! I do my Kegel's every day," replied Doris. "And, by the way, I keep the porta-potties on my job sites very clean...not that I would eat off the floor or anything, but...I do look out for my employees." Doris defined her life through the thing she loved most in life—... her work.

On physical examination, Doris was afebrile. Her respirations were 18 and her pulse was 74 and regular. Her blood pressure was slightly elevated at 142/84. I made a note to recheck it again before she left because who knew when or if she would come back. Her head, ears, eyes, nose, and throat (HEENT) examination was normal, as was her cardiopulmonary examination. Her abdominal examination revealed no abnormal mass or organomegaly. There was no costovertebral angle (CVA) tenderness. There was no peripheral edema. Palpation of the lumbar paraspinous muscles revealed tenderness to deep palpation and significant spasm of the paraspinous muscles, the right greater than the left.

SENSORY

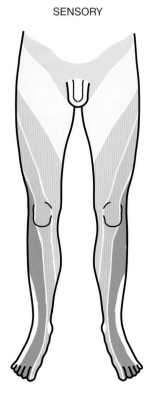

Fig. 11.1 Sensory distribution of the L5 dermatome (turquoise). (From Waldman SD. *Physical Diagnosis of Pain: An Atlas of Signs and Symptoms*. 3rd ed. St. Louis: Elsevier; 2016: Fig. 145.1.)

I asked Doris to stand up. Her balance was fine, but she had limited range of motion of the lumbar spine with flexion, extension, and lateral bending. I asked Doris which movement caused the most pain and she indicated extension and left lateral bending. Doris was able to toe walk without difficulty, but she had lots of trouble with the right leg when I asked her to walk on her heels. "The right foot feels weak," she volunteered.

A careful neurologic examination of the lower extremities revealed a normal sensory examination on the left, but decreased sensation over the dorsum of the foot and between the great and second toe on the right (Fig. 11.1). I asked her to lift up her toes against my hand as hard as she could and to try and push my hand away. Her left side was fine, but her extensor hallucis longus was quite weak on the right (Fig. 11.2). Her knee jerk and ankle jerk reflexes were physiologic bilaterally. Doris's upper extremity motor and sensory examination, as well as upper extremity deep tendon reflexes, were normal. The Lasegue test was positive on the right (Fig. 11.3). No pathologic reflexes or clonus were identified.

MOTOR

L5

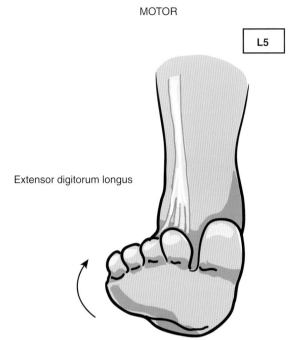

Extensor digitorum longus

Fig. 11.2 L5 manual muscle testing. (From Waldman SD. *Physical Diagnosis of Pain: An Atlas of Signs and Symptoms*. 3rd ed. St. Louis: Elsevier; 2016, Fig. 145.2.)

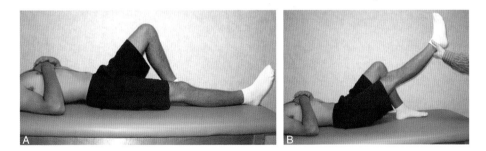

Fig. 11.3 Lasegue sign testing. (A) The Lasegue straight leg raising test: The patient is in the supine position with the unaffected leg flexed to 45 degrees at the knee and the affected leg placed flat against the table. (B) The Lasegue straight leg raising test: With the ankle of the affected leg placed at 90 degrees of flexion, the affected leg is slowly raised toward the ceiling while the knee is kept fully extended. (From Waldman SD. *Physical Diagnosis of Pain: An Atlas of Signs and Symptoms*. 3rd ed. St. Louis: Elsevier; 2016: Fig. 147.2.)

Key Clinical Points—What's Important and What's Not

THE HISTORY

- No history of acute trauma
- Weak history of previous back pain
- Back pain radiating from the low back into the right lower extremity
- Sensation that right leg "wanted to buckle"
- Numbness down the back of the leg and into the dorsum of the foot
- Difficulty climbing a ladder
- No bowel or bladder symptomatology

THE PHYSICAL EXAMINATION

- The patient is afebrile
- Decreased sensation down the back of the leg and into the dorsum of the foot (see Fig. 11.1)
- Weakness of the extensor hallucis longus on the right (see Fig. 11.2)
- Inability to heel walk, consistent with weakness of the L5 innervated muscles
- Normal left upper and lower extremity motor and sensory examination
- No pathologic reflexes
- No clonus
- Positive Lasegue sign bilaterally (see Fig. 11.3)

OTHER FINDINGS OF NOTE

- Normal HEENT examination
- Normal cardiovascular examination
- Normal pulmonary examination
- Normal abdominal examination
- No peripheral edema

What Tests Would You Like to Order?

The following tests were ordered:
- Plain radiographs, lumbar spine
- Magnetic resonance imaging (MRI) of the lumbar spine
- Electromyography and nerve conduction velocity testing of the low back and right lower extremities

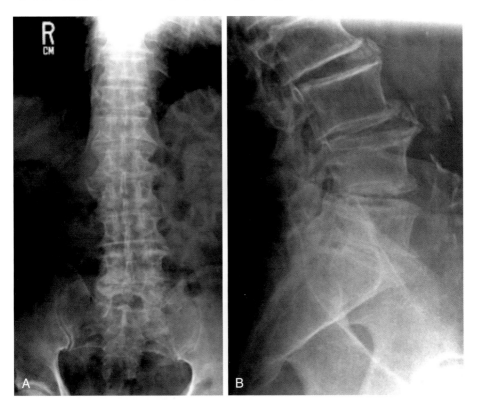

Fig. 11.4   Lumbar spondylosis. Anteroposterior (A) and lateral (B) radiographs of the lumbar spine show the cardinal features of disc space narrowing, marginal osteophytes, and endplate sclerosis. (Courtesy Dr. John Crues, University of California, San Diego.)

TEST RESULTS

The plain radiographs revealed disk space narrowing, marginal osteo-phytes, and endplate sclerosis, consistent with lumbar spondylosis (Fig. 11.4). The MRI scan of Doris's lumbar spine revealed significant lumbar spondylosis (Fig. 11.5). The electromyogram was positive for acute denervation of the L5 innervated muscles on the right. Nerve con-duction velocity test revealed no evidence of entrapment or peripheral neuropathy.

📋 Clinical Correlation—Putting It All Together

What is the diagnosis?

- L5 radiculopathy on right secondary to lumbar spondylosis

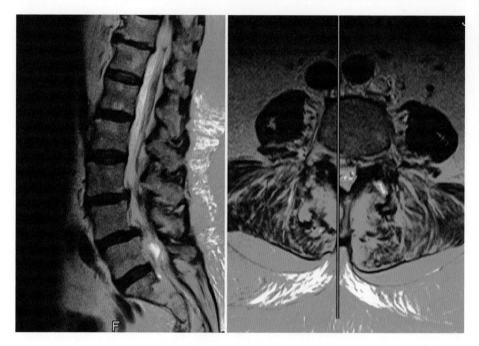

Fig. 11.5 Magnetic resonance image (MRI) of the lumbar spine, revealing lumbar spondylosis. (From Yue J, Guyer R, Johnson JP, Khoo L, Hochschuler S. *The Comprehensive Treatment of the Aging Spine*. Philadelphia: Saunders; 2011: Fig. 13.1.)

The Science Behind the Diagnosis

THE DERMATOMES AND MYOTOMES

The innervation of the skin, muscles, and deep structures in humans is determined embryologically at an early stage of fetal development, and there is amazingly little intersubject variability. Each segment of the spinal cord and its corresponding spinal nerves have a consistent segmental relationship that allows the clinician to ascertain the probable spinal level of dysfunction based on the pattern of pain, muscle weakness, and deep tendon reflex changes.

In general, in humans, the more proximal the muscle, the more cephalad is the spinal segment, with the ventral muscles innervated by higher spinal segments than the corresponding dorsal muscles (Figs. 11.6 and 11.7). Pain perceived in the region of a given muscle or joint may not be coming from the muscle or joint, but simply be referred by problems at the same lumbar spinal segment that innervates the muscles. Furthermore, the clinician needs to be aware that the relative consistent pattern of dermatomal and myotomal distribution breaks down when the pain is perceived in the deep structures of the upper extremity (e.g., the joints and tendinous insertions). With pain in these regions, the clinician should refer to a sclerotomal chart.

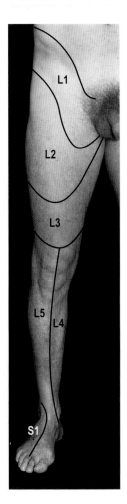

Fig. 11.6 Dermatomes of the lower extremity—Anterior view. (From Jacob S. *Human Anatomy*. Philadelphia: Churchill Livingstone; 2008: Fig. 6.92.)

The concept of diagnosing a problem at a specific neurologic level via physical examination has its basis in the fact that pathology at the lumbar spinal cord or lumbar nerve root level manifests itself in a relatively consistent manner by dysfunction, numbness, and pain of the upper extremity, which occurs in a dermatomal distribution. Although not foolproof, a careful physical examination of the upper extremity with an eye to the neurologic level affected can frequently guide the clinician in designing a more targeted workup and treatment plan. By overlapping the information gleaned from physical examination with the neuroanatomic information gained from MRI and the neurophysiologic information from electromyography, a highly

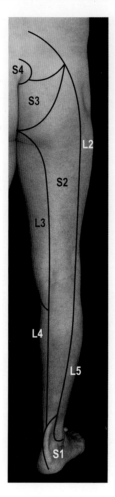

Fig. 11.7 Dermatomes of the lower extremity—Posterior view. (From Jacob S. *Human Anatomy*. Philadelphia: Churchill Livingstone; 2008: Fig. 6.93.)

accurate diagnosis can be made as to what level of the lumbar spine is responsible for the patient's symptoms.

Testing for the L5 dermatome is best carried out by a careful sensory evaluation of the skin overlying the dorsum of the foot of the affected lower extremity (see Fig. 11.1). Decreased sensation in this anatomic region can be ascribed to proximal lesions of the spinal cord, such as a spinal cord tumor or multiple sclerosis; to more distal lesions of the L5 nerve root, such as impingement by a herniated disc; or to a lesion of the more peripheral axillary nerve (Fig. 11.8). For this reason, correlation with manual muscle testing and evaluation of the deep tendon reflex combined with radiographic and electromyographic testing can help to determine the exact site of the pathology (Table 11.1).

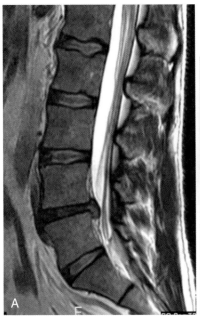
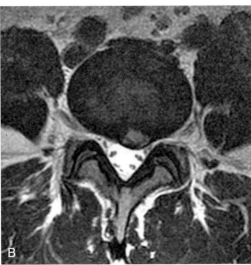

Fig. 11.8 Lumbar disk extrusion. (A) The sagittal T2-weighted magnetic resonance image shows an extruded disc at the L4-5 level. (B) The axial image through the L4-L5 level shows disc extrusion to the left side of the neural canal, which is compressing the exiting L5 nerve root against the left lamina. (Courtesy Dr. John Crues, University of California, San Diego.)

TABLE 11.1 ■ **Clinical Features of Lumbar Radiculopathy**

Lumbar Root	Pain	Sensory Changes	Weakness	Reflex Changes
L4 root	Back, shin, thigh, leg	Shin numbness	Ankle dorsiflexors	Knee jerk
L5 root	Back, posterior thigh, leg	Numbness, top of foot and first web space	Extensor hallucis longus	None
S1 root	Back, posterior calf, leg	Numbness, lateral foot	Gastrocnemius and soleus	Ankle jerk

Testing for the L5 myotome is best carried out by manual muscle testing of the extensor hallucis longus. This muscle is primarily innervated by the L5 spinal nerve. Because in most patients, the extensor function of the extensor hallucis longus of the foot is an L5 function, the muscle should be tested as follows: The patient is placed in the sitting position on the examination table. The examiner then puts downward pressure on the big toe of the affected side and then asks the patient to lift the toe up to push the examiner's hand away (see Fig. 11.2). If the manual muscle testing is normal, the examiner should not be able to resist the patient's ability to extend the great toe.

LUMBAR RADICULOPATHY

Lumbar radiculopathy is a constellation of symptoms consisting of neurogenic back and lower extremity pain emanating from the lumbar nerve roots. In addition to the pain, the patient with lumbar radiculopathy may experience associated numbness, weakness, and loss of reflexes. The causes of lumbar radiculopathy include herniated disc, foraminal stenosis, tumor, osteophyte formation, and rarely, infection (Table 11.2). Many patients and their physicians will use the term sciatica to refer to the constellation of symptoms known as lumbar radiculopathy.

SIGNS AND SYMPTOMS

The patient suffering from lumbar radiculopathy will complain of pain, numbness, tingling, and paresthesias in the distribution of the affected nerve root or

TABLE 11.2 ■ Clinical Syndromes That Can Mimic Low Back Pain and Lumbar Radiculopathy

Localized Bony, Disc Space, or Joint Space Pathology	Primary Hip Pathology	Systemic Disease	Sympathetically Mediated Pain	Pain Referred from Other Body Areas
Vertebral fracture	Bursitis	Rheumatoid	Causalgia	Pancreatitis
Primary bone tumor	Tendinitis	arthritis	Reflex sympathetic	Malignancy of the
Facet joint disease	Aseptic	Collagen vascular	dystrophy	retroperitoneal
Localized or gener-	necrosis	disease	Postthrombophlebitis	space
alized degener-	Osteoarthritis	Reiter syndrome	pain (milk leg)	Lumbar
ative arthritis	Joint instability	Gout		Plexopathy
Osteophyte	Muscle strain	Other crystal		Fibromyalgia
formation	Muscle sprain	arthropathies		Myofascial pain
Disc space	Periarticular	Charcot neuro-		syndromes
infection	infection	pathic arthritis		Entrapment
Herniated lumbar	not involv-	Multiple sclerosis		neuropathies
disc	ing joint	Ischemic pain		Intraabdominal
Degenerative disc	space	secondary to		tumors
disease		peripheral		
Primary spinal cord		vascular		
and/or cauda		insufficiency		
equina		Ankylosing		
pathology		spondylitis		
Osteomyelitis				
Epidural abcess				
Epidural hematoma				

From Waldman SD. *Physical Diagnosis of Pain: An Atlas of Signs and Symptoms*. 3rd ed. St. Louis: Elsevier; 2016: Table 137.1.

roots (see Table 11.1). Patients may also note weakness and lack of coordination in the affected extremity. Muscle spasms and back pain, as well as pain referred into the buttocks, are common. Decreased sensation, weakness, and reflex changes are demonstrated on physical examination. Patients with lumbar radiculopathy will commonly experience a reflex shifting of the trunk to one side. This reflex shifting is called a lateral shift or a list. Occasionally, a patient suffering from lumbar radiculopathy will experience compression of the lumbar spinal nerve roots and cauda equina, resulting in myelopathy or cauda equina syndrome. Lumbar myelopathy is most commonly caused by a midline herniated lumbar disc, spinal stenosis, tumor, or rarely, infection. Patients suffering from lumbar myelopathy or cauda equina syndrome will experience varying degrees of lower extremity weakness and bowel and bladder symptomatology. This represents a neurosurgical emergency and should be treated as such.

TESTING

Magnetic resonance imaging of the lumbar spine will provide the clinician with the best information regarding the lumbar spine and its contents. MRI is highly accurate and will help identify abnormalities that may put the patient at risk for the development of lumbar myelopathy (see Figs. 11.8 and 11.9). In patients who cannot undergo MRI (e.g., patients with a pacemaker), computed tomography or myelography is a reasonable second choice and may further elucidate bony abnormalities (Fig. 11.10). Discography may provide additional useful information in selected cases (Fig. 11.11). Radionuclide bone scanning and plain radiographs are indicated if fracture or a bony abnormality, such as metastatic disease, is being considered. Although this testing provides the clinician with useful neuroanatomic information, electromyography and nerve conduction velocity testing will provide the clinician with neurophysiologic information that can delineate the actual status of each nerve root and the lumbar plexus. Screening laboratory testing consisting of complete blood count, erythrocyte sedimentation rate, and automated blood chemistry testing should be performed if the diagnosis of lumbar radiculopathy is in question.

DIFFERENTIAL DIAGNOSIS

Lumbar radiculopathy is a clinical diagnosis that is supported by a combination of clinical history, physical examination, radiography, and MRI. Pain syndromes that may mimic lumbar radiculopathy include low back strain, lumbar bursitis, lumbar fibromyositis, inflammatory arthritis, and disorders of the lumbar spinal cord, roots, plexus, and nerves (see Table 11.2). MRI of the lumbar spine should be carried out on all patients suspected of suffering from lumbar radiculopathy. Screening laboratory testing consisting of complete blood count, erythrocyte sedimentation rate, antinuclear antibody testing, HLA-B27 antigen screening, and

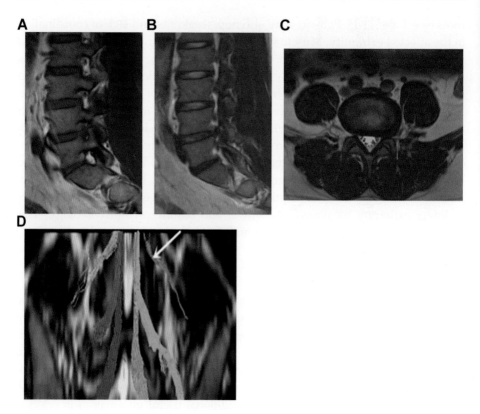

Fig. 11.9 Sagittal T1-weighted imaging (A), sagittal T2-weighted imaging (B), and axial T2-weighted imaging (C) reveal left posterolateral prolapse of intervertebral disc at L4-L5 and compression of ipsilateral L4 nerve root in a 56-year-old woman. Fiber tractography (D) shows compression of ipsilateral L4 nerve root (*arrow*) on color-coded diffusion tensor imaging and fiber tractography images. (From He A, Wang W-Z, Qiao P-F, Qiao G-Y, Cheng H, Feng P-Y. Quantitative evaluation of compressed L4-5 and S1 nerve roots of lumbar disc herniation patients by diffusion tensor imaging and fiber tractography. *World Neurosurg.* 2018;115:e45–e52; Fig. 3.)

automated blood chemistry testing should be performed if the diagnosis of lumbar radiculopathy is in question to help rule out other causes of the patient's pain.

THE INTERVERTEBRAL DISC

The lumbar intervertebral disc has two major functions. The first is to serve as the major shock-absorbing structure of the lumbar spine, and the second is to facilitate the synchronized movement of the lumbar spine while helping to prevent impingement of the neural structures and vasculature that traverse the lumbar spine. Both the shock-absorbing function and the movement/protective function of the lumbar intervertebral disc are functions of the disc structure as well as of the laws of physics that affect it.

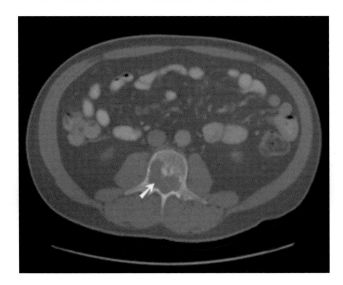

Fig. 11.10 Axial computed tomography (CT) image in bone window shows a central destructive lesion in the body of the L3 vertebra (*arrow*). (From Hatem MA. Lumbar spine chordoma. *Radiol Case Rep.* 2014;9(3):940, Fig. 1.)

To understand how the lumbar intervertebral disc functions in health and becomes dysfunctional in disease, it is useful to think of the disc as a closed, fluid-filled container. The outside of the container is made up of a top and bottom, called the endplates, which are composed of relatively inflexible hyaline cartilage. The sides of the lumbar intervertebral disc are made up of a woven crisscrossing matrix of fibroelastic fibers that tightly attaches to the top and bottom endplates. This woven matrix of fibers is called the annulus, and it completely surrounds the sides of the disc (see Fig. 3.5). The interlaced structure of the annulus results in an enclosing mesh that is extremely strong yet very flexible, which facilitates the compression of the disc during the wide range of motion of the lumbar spine (see Fig. 3.6).

Inside this container consisting of the top and bottom endplates and surrounding annulus is the water-containing mucopolysaccharide gel-like substance called the nucleus pulposus (see Fig. 10.12A). The nucleus is incompressible and transmits any pressure placed on one portion of the disc to the surrounding nucleus. In health, the water-filled gel creates a positive intradiscal pressure, which forces apart the adjacent vertebra and helps protect the spinal cord and exiting nerve roots. When the lumbar spine moves, the incompressible nature of the nucleus pulposus maintains a constant intradiscal pressure while some fibers of the disc relax and others contract.

As the lumbar intervertebral disc ages, it becomes less vascular and loses its ability to absorb water into the disc (see Fig. 10.12B-D). This

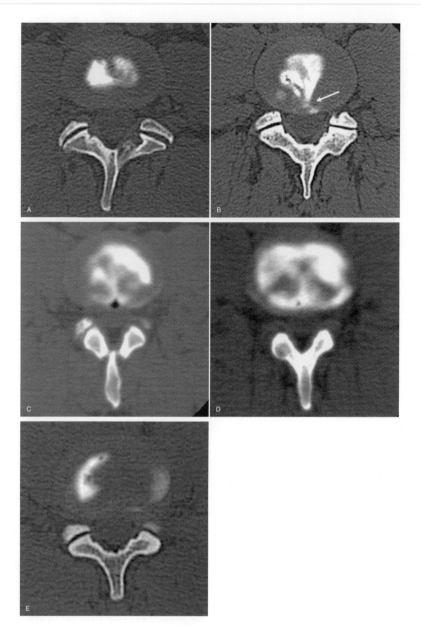

Fig. 11.11 Computed tomography (CT) characterization after intradiscal contrast injection: post-discography transaxial CT images. (A) Normal nucleogram characterized by a central globule of contrast material that remains within the expected confines of the nucleus pulposus. (B) Annular fissure. Contrast material is noted within the nucleus pulposus, but it also extends in radial fashion posteriorly beyond the expected confines of the nucleus pulposus into the region of the annulus fibrosus (*arrow*). (C) Annular tear with protrusion. (D) Degenerative disk disease with irregular and disorganized contrast within the nucleus and inner annulus. (E) Annular injection. Contrast material is seen only in a small circumferential pattern along the inner annulus without any central contrast accumulation. Such an annular injection could cause a false-positive pain response at provocation discography. (From Waldman SD, Bloch J. *Pain Management*. Philadelphia: Saunders; 2007, Fig. 9.4.)

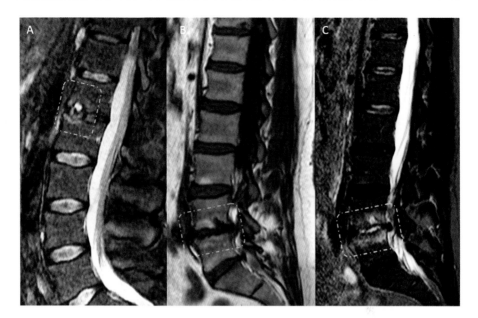

Fig. 11.12 Schmorl's nodes with T2-weighted magnetic resonance imaging showing edematous change. (A) T2-weighted image shows painful Schmorl's node at L1. (B and C) T1-weighted image and fat-suppressed T2-weighted image (STIR) show type 1 modic change at L5/S1. and edematous Schmorl's node. Both patients had back pain. *STIR,* Short tau inversion recovery. (From Xiáng YXJ, Wu A-M, Santiago FR, Nogueira-Barbosa MH. Informed appropriate imaging for low back pain management: a narrative review. *J Orthop Transl.* 2018;15, Fig. 3.)

results in degradation of the disc's shock-absorbing and motion-facilitating functions. This problem worsens by degeneration of the annulus, which allows portions of the disc wall to bulge, distorting the ability of the nucleus pulposus to distribute evenly the forces placed on it throughout the entire disc. This exacerbates disc dysfunction and can contribute to further disc deterioration, which may ultimately lead to actual complete disruption of the annulus and extrusion of the nucleus. Intervertebral discs may herniate laterally, posteriorly, and anteriorly as well as superiorly or inferiorly through weakened vertebral endplates (Fig. 11.12). This deterioration of the disc is responsible for many of the painful conditions emanating from the lumbar spine that are encountered in clinical practice.

MANAGEMENT AND TREATMENT

Lumbar radiculopathy is best treated with a multimodality approach. Physical therapy, including heat modalities and deep sedative massage, combined with nonsteroidal antiinflammatory agents and skeletal muscle relaxants, represents a reasonable starting point. The addition of caudal or

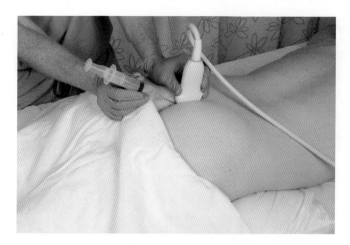

Fig. 11.13   Ultrasound-guided caudal epidural block. (From Waldman SD. *Atlas of Interventional Pain Management*. 4th ed. Philadelphia: Saunders; 2015, Fig. 105.23.)

lumbar steroid epidural nerve blocks is a reasonable next step (Fig. 11.13). Caudal or lumbar epidural blocks with local anesthetic and steroid have been shown to be extremely effective in the treatment of lumbar radiculopathy. Underlying sleep disturbance and depression are best treated with a tricyclic antidepressant compound such as nortriptyline, which can be started at a single bedtime dose of 25 mg.

HIGH-YIELD TAKEAWAYS

- The patient is afebrile, making an acute infectious etiology (e.g., epidural abscess) unlikely.
- The patient's symptomatology is the result of acute trauma to the lumbar intervertebral disc.
- The patient's pain is localized in the back and right lower extremity, which is highly suggestive of lumbar radiculopathy.
- The patient's symptoms are unilateral, which would be more suggestive of lumbar radiculopathy vs. other pathologic processes, although bilateral radiculopathy is not that uncommon.
- The patient's neurologic examination is abnormal in the affected right lower extremity with L4 sensory deficit, ankle dorsiflexor weakness, and a diminished knee jerk reflex, which is highly suggestive of a right L4 radiculopathy.
- There are no bowel or bladder symptoms or pathologic reflexes suggestive of myelopathy.
- MRI scanning is highly sensitive in the diagnosis of discogenic disease and is useful in ruling out other space-occupying lesions that may be producing radicular symptoms (see Figs. 10.5 and 10.9).

Suggested Readings

Barr K. Electrodiagnosis of lumbar radiculopathy. *Phys Med Rehabil Clin N Am*. 2013;24 (1):79–91.

Waldman SD. Functional anatomy of the lumbar spine. In: *Physical Diagnosis of Pain: An Atlas of Signs and Symptoms*. 4th ed. Philadelphia: Elsevier; 2020.

Waldman SD. Lumbar radiculopathy. In: *Pain Review*. 2nd ed. Philadelphia: Elsevier; 2017:256–257.

Waldman SD. Lumbar epidural nerve block: Interlaminar approach. In: *Atlas of Interventional Pain Management*. 4th ed. Philadelphia: Elsevier; 2015:500–513.

Waldman SD. The Lesegue straight leg raiding test for lumbar radiculopathy. In: *Physical Diagnosis of Pain: An Atlas of Signs and Symptoms*. 3rd ed. Philadelphia: Elsevier; 2016:235–236.

Waldman SD, Campbell RSD. Anatomy: Special imaging considerations of the lumbar spine. In: *Imaging of Pain*. Philadelphia: Elsevier; 2011:109–110.

Amy Turner

A 28-Year-Old Female With Severe Low Back Pain That Radiates Into the Right Calf

- Learn the common causes of lumbar radiculopathy.
- Develop an understanding of the role of the intervertebral disc in lumbar radiculopathy.
- Develop an understanding of the causes of lumbar radiculopathy.
- Learn the clinical presentation of lumbar radiculopathy.
- Learn how to use physical examination to determine which lumbar spinal nerve roots are subserving the patient's pain.
- Learn to distinguish lumbar strain from lumbar radiculopathy.
- Learn the important anatomic structures in lumbar radiculopathy.
- Develop an understanding of the treatment options for lumbar radiculopathy.
- Learn the appropriate testing options to help diagnose lumbar radiculopathy.
- Learn to identify red flags waving in patients who present with lumbar radiculopathy.
- Develop an understanding of the role in interventional pain management in the treatment of lumbar radiculopathy.

Amy Turner

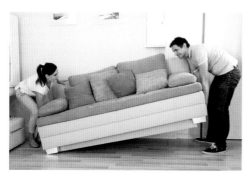

Amy Turner is a 28-year-old graphic designer with the chief complaint of "searing, white-hot pain across my low back and hat shoots down from my back into the calf of my right leg." The pain began when Amy decided that she wanted to move her sofa to the opposite side of the living room. She enlisted the help of her husband, Chad. "Chad made me pick up the heavy end of the sofa…the one that was up close to the TV…so that made it hard to get under the sofa to pick it up. I lifted funny and all of sudden, I felt something give in my back. There was a sudden searing, white-hot pain across my low back and the pain shot down from my back into the calf of my right leg. It hurt really bad, so, I dropped my end of the sofa…which caused Chad to drop his end." For the past 3 weeks, Amy had tried to tough it out—…"tried all the usual stuff…tea tree oil, Motrin, the heating pad…Chad wanted me to go to the chiropractor, but I was afraid it might make my back worse."

I asked Amy to point with one finger where it hurts the most. Amy pointed to her lower lumbar spine and then pointed all the way down the back of her right leg. "Is there any numbness?" I asked. Amy replied that the side of her right foot had a weird pins and needles feeling that got worse when she sat at her drafting table for long periods of time. "Are you having any problem peeing or pooping?" I asked. "For the last week or so, I have really been dreading going to the bathroom, because when I bear down, it causes the pain to shoot down my leg. I just started my period and that made my back hurt worse."

On physical examination, Amy Turner was afebrile and her respirations were 16. Her pulse was 74 and regular with a blood pressure of 110/68. Her head, ears, eyes, nose, and throat (HEENT) examination was normal, as was her cardiopulmonary examination. Her abdominal examination revealed no abnormal mass or organomegaly. There was no costovertebral angle (CVA) tenderness. There was no peripheral edema. Palpation of the lumbar paraspinous muscles revealed tenderness to deep palpation and significant spasm of the paraspinous muscles, the right greater than the left.

I asked Amy to stand up and walk for me. Her balance was fine, but she had limited range of motion of the lumbar spine with flexion,

SENSORY

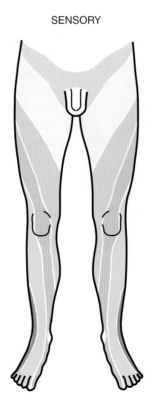

Fig. 12.1   Sensory distribution of the S1 dermatome (*orange*). (From Waldman SD. *Physical Diagnosis of Pain: An Atlas of Signs and Symptoms*. 3rd ed. St. Louis: Elsevier; 2016: Fig. 146.1.)

extension, and lateral bending. Amy was able to heel walk without diffi-culty, but she had lots of trouble with the right leg when I asked her to walk on her toes. "The toes on my right foot won't work," she volun-teered. I reassured her that she was doing fine and that I wanted her to sit back up on the examination table so I could check her reflexes.

A careful neurologic examination of the lower extremities revealed a normal sensory examination on the left, but decreased sensation over the lateral side of the foot on the right (Fig. 12.1). I pushed against the lateral sides of her feet and asked her to try and push my hands away. Her left side was fine, but she had almost no foot eversion on the right (Fig. 12.2). Her knee jerk reflexes were normal bilaterally, as was her ankle jerk reflex on the left, but the right ankle jerk was completely absent (Fig. 12.3). Amy's upper extremity motor and sensory examination, as well as her upper extremity deep tendon reflexes, were normal. The Lasegue test was markedly positive on the right, with Amy crying out in pain as I lifted her right leg (Fig. 12.4). No pathologic reflexes or clonus were identified.

MOTOR

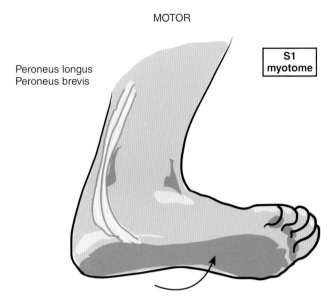

Peroneus longus
Peroneus brevis

S1
myotome

Fig. 12.2 S1 manual muscle testing. (From Waldman SD. *Physical Diagnosis of Pain: An Atlas of Signs and Symptoms*. 3rd ed. St. Louis: Elsevier; 2016: Fig. 146.2.)

REFLEX

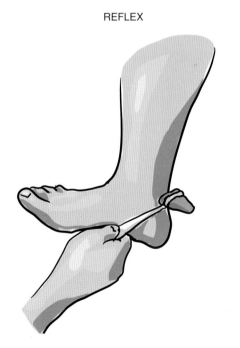

Fig. 12.3 Ankle jerk deep tendon reflex. (From Waldman SD. *Physical Diagnosis of Pain: An Atlas of Signs and Symptoms*. 3rd ed. St. Louis: Elsevier; 2016: Fig. 146.3.)

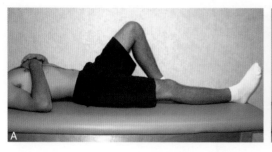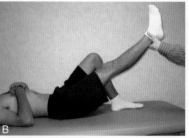

Fig. 12.4   The Lasegue straight leg raising test. (A) The patient is in the supine position with the unaffected leg flexed to 45 degrees at the knee and the affected leg placed flat against the table. (B) With the ankle of the affected leg placed at 90 degrees of flexion, the affected leg is slowly raised toward the ceiling while the knee is kept fully extended. (From Waldman SD. *Physical Diagnosis of Pain: An Atlas of Signs and Symptoms*. 3rd ed. St. Louis: Elsevier; 2016: Figs. 147.1 and 147.2.)

Key Clinical Points—What's Important and What's Not

THE HISTORY

- History of acute trauma when lifting a heavy sofa
- No history of previous back pain
- Back pain radiating from the low back into the right lower extremity
- Numbness down the back of the leg and into the side of the foot
- Difficulty sitting for long periods of time
- No bowel or bladder symptomatology

THE PHYSICAL EXAMINATION

- The patient is afebrile
- Decreased sensation down the back of the leg and into the lateral aspect of the foot see Fig. 12.1)
- Weakness of the ankle everters on the right (see Fig. 12.2)
- Inability to toe walk consistent with weakness of the S1 innervated muscles
- Normal upper extremity motor and sensory examination
- Absent ankle jerk on the right (see Fig. 12.3)
- No pathologic reflexes
- No clonus
- Positive Lasegue sign bilaterally (see Fig. 12.4)

OTHER FINDINGS OF NOTE

- Normal HEENT examination
- Normal cardiovascular examination

- Normal pulmonary examination
- Normal abdominal examination
- No peripheral edema

What Tests Would You Like to Order?

The following tests were ordered:
- Magnetic resonance imaging (MRI) of the lumbar spine
- Electromyogram and nerve conduction studies of the right lower extremity

TEST RESULTS

The MRI scan of Amy Turner's lumbar spine revealed a large L5/S1 disc extrusion causing compression of the theca and nerve root. There was enhancement of the swollen nerve root. Complicating the picture was disc bulging at L4-L5 and a torn annulus at L5-S1 (Fig. 12.5) The electromyogram was positive for significant acute denervation of the S1 innervated muscles on the right. Nerve conduction velocity test revealed no evidence of entrapment or peripheral neuropathy.

Clinical Correlation—Putting It All Together

What is the diagnosis?
- S1 radiculopathy on right secondary to herniated vertebral disc

The Science Behind the Diagnosis

THE DERMATOMES AND MYOTOMES

Innervation of the skin, muscles, and deep structures in humans is determined embryologically at an early stage of fetal development, and there is amazingly little intersubject variability. Each segment of the spinal cord and its corresponding spinal nerves have a consistent segmental relationship that allows the clinician to ascertain the probable spinal level of dysfunction based on the pattern of pain, muscle weakness, and deep tendon reflex changes.

In general, in humans, the more proximal the muscle, the more cephalad is the spinal segment, with the ventral muscles innervated by higher spinal segments than the corresponding dorsal muscles (Figs. 12.6 and 12.7). Pain perceived in the region of a given muscle or joint may not be coming from the muscle or joint, but simply be referred by problems at the same lumbar spinal segment that innervates the muscles. Furthermore, the clinician needs to be aware that the

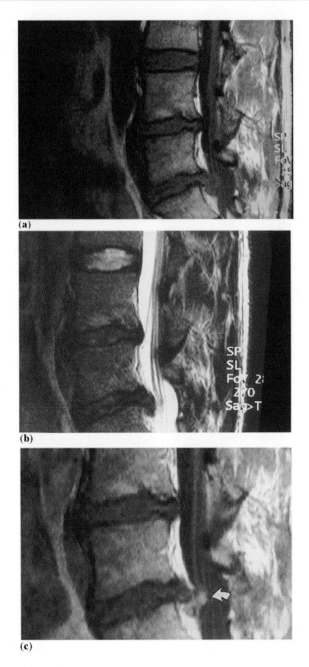

Fig. 12.5 Magnetic resonance image (MRI) of the lumbar spine. Sagittal T1 spin-echo (A), T2 fast spin-echo (B), and post-gadolinium T1 spin-echo (C) images of a large L5/S1 disc extrusion causing compression of the theca and nerve root. Note the perifocal disc and swollen nerve root enhancement (*arrow*). The L5/S1 annulus is torn and the L4/L5 level bulges. (From Cassar-Pullicino VN. MRI of the ageing and herniating intervertebral disc. *Eur J Radiol.* 1998;27(3):214−228, Fig. 6.)

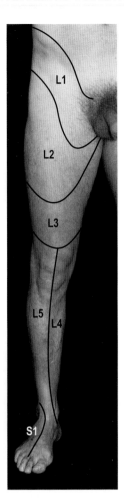

Fig. 12.6 Dermatomes of the lower extremity—Anterior view. (From Jacob S. *Human Anatomy.* Churchill Livingstone; 2008: Fig. 6.92.)

relative consistent pattern of dermatomal and myotomal distribution breaks down when the pain is perceived in the deep structures of the upper extremity (e.g., the joints and tendinous insertions). With pain in these regions, the clinician should refer to a sclerotomal chart.

The concept of diagnosing a problem at a specific neurologic level via physical examination has its basis in the fact that pathology at the lumbar spinal cord or lumbar nerve root level manifests itself in a relatively consistent manner by dysfunction, numbness, and pain of the upper extremity, which occurs in a dermatomal distribution. Although not foolproof, a careful physical examination of the upper extremity with an eye to the neurologic level affected can frequently guide the clinician in designing a more targeted workup and treatment plan. By

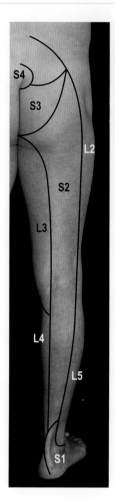

Fig. 12.7 Dermatomes of the lower extremity—Posterior view. (From Jacob S. *Human Anatomy.* Churchill Livingstone; 2008: Fig. 6.93.)

overlapping the information gleaned from physical examination with the neuro-anatomic information gained from magnetic resonance imaging and the neurophysiologic information from electromyography, a highly accurate diagnosis can be made as to what level of the lumbar spine is responsible for the patient's symptoms.

Testing for the S1 dermatome is best carried out by a careful sensory evaluation of the skin overlying the lateral aspect of the foot of the affected lower extremity (see Fig. 12.1). Decreased sensation in this anatomic region can be ascribed to proximal lesions of the spinal cord, such as a spinal cord tumor or multiple sclerosis; to more distal lesions of the S1 nerve root, such as impingement by a herniated disc; or to a lesion of the more

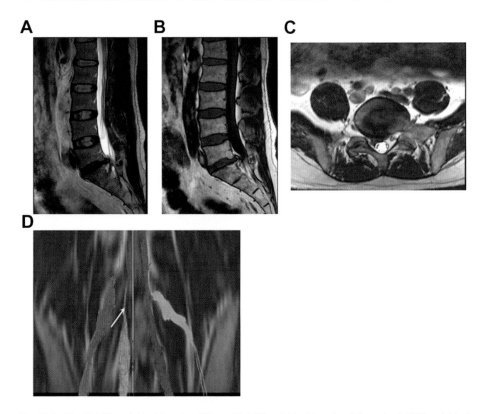

Fig. 12.8   Sagittal T1-weighted imaging (A), sagittal T2-weighted imaging (B), and axial T2-weighted imaging (C) show prolapse of intervertebral disc at L5-S1 in a 38-year-old man. Fiber tractography (D) shows compression of the right spinal root at L5-S1 (*arrow*) on color-coded diffusion tensor imaging and fiber tractography images. (From He A, Wang W-Z, Qiao P-F, Qiao G-Y, Cheng H, Feng P-Y. Quantitative evaluation of compressed L4-5 and S1 nerve roots of lumbar disc herniation patients by diffusion tensor imaging and fiber tractography. *World Neurosurg*. 2018;115:e45–e52, Fig. 2.)

peripheral axillary nerve (Fig. 12.8). For this reason, correlation with manual muscle testing and evaluation of the deep tendon reflex combined with radiographic and electromyographic testing can help to determine the exact site of pathology (Table 12.1).

Testing for the S1 myotome is best carried out by manual muscle testing of the ankle everters as well as the gastrocnemius and soleus muscles. These muscles are primarily innervated by the S1 spinal nerve. Because, in most patients, the ankle eversion function of these muscles is a S1 function, the muscle should be tested as follows: The patient is placed in the sitting position on the examination table. The examiner then puts his or her hand on the outside of the foot and pushes inward. The patient is then asked to push the examiner's hand away by everting the ankle (see Fig. 12.2). If the manual muscle testing is normal, the examiner should not be able to resist the patient's ability to extend the great toe.

TABLE 12.1 ■ **Clinical Features of Lumbar Radiculopathy**

Lumbar Root	Pain	Sensory Changes	Weakness	Reflex Changes
L4 root	Back, shin, thigh, leg	Shin numbness	Ankle dorsiflexors	Knee jerk
L5 root	Back, posterior thigh, leg	Numbness top of foot and first web space	Extensor hallucis longus	None
S1 root	Back, posterior calf, leg	Numbness lateral foot	Gastrocnemius and soleus	Ankle jerk

TABLE 12.2 ■ **Clinical Syndromes That Can Mimic Low Back Pain and Lumbar Radiculopathy**

Localized Bony, Disc Space, or Joint Space Pathology	Primary Hip Pathology	Systemic Disease	Sympathetically Mediated Pain	Pain Referred from Other Body Areas
Vertebral fracture	Bursitis	Rheumatoid arthritis	Causalgia	Pancreatitis
Primary bone tumor	Tendinitis	Collagen vascular disease	Reflex sympathetic dystrophy	Malignancy of the retroperitoneal space
Facet joint disease	Aseptic necrosis	Reiter syndrome	Postthrombophlebitis pain (milk leg)	Lumbar plexopathy
Localized or generalized degenerative arthritis	Osteoarthritis	Gout		Fibromyalgia
Osteophyte formation	Joint instability	Other crystal arthropathies		Myofascial pain syndromes
Disc space infection	Muscle strain	Charcot neuropathic arthritis		Entrapment neuropathies
Herniated lumbar disc	Muscle sprain	Multiple sclerosis		Intraabdominal tumors
Degenerative disc disease	Periarticular infection not involving joint space	Ischemic pain secondary to peripheral vascular insufficiency		
Primary spinal cord and/or cauda equina pathology		Ankylosing spondylitis		
Osteomyelitis				
Epidural abscess				
Epidural hematoma				

From Waldman SD. *Physical Diagnosis of Pain: An Atlas of Signs and Symptoms.* 3rd ed. St. Louis: Elsevier; 2016: Table 137.1.

LUMBAR RADICULOPATHY

Lumbar radiculopathy is a constellation of symptoms consisting of neurogenic back and lower extremity pain emanating from the lumbar nerve roots. In addition to the pain, the patient with lumbar radiculopathy may experience associated numbness, weakness, and loss of reflexes. The causes of lumbar radiculopathy include herniated disc, foraminal stenosis, tumor, osteophyte formation, and rarely, infection (Table 12.2). Many patients and their physicians will use the term *sciatica* to refer to the constellation of symptoms known as lumbar radiculopathy.

SIGNS AND SYMPTOMS

The patient suffering from lumbar radiculopathy will complain of pain, numbness, tingling, and paresthesias in the distribution of the affected nerve root or roots (see Table 12.1). Patients may also note weakness and lack of coordination in the affected extremity. Muscle spasms and back pain, as well as pain referred into the buttocks, are common. Decreased sensation, weakness, and reflex changes are demonstrated on physical examination. Patients with lumbar radiculopathy will commonly experience a reflex shifting of the trunk to one side. This reflex shifting is called a lateral shift or a list. Occasionally a patient suffering from lumbar radiculopathy will experience compression of the lumbar spinal nerve roots and cauda equina, resulting in myelopathy or cauda equina syndrome. Lumbar myelopathy is most commonly caused by a midline herniated lumbar disc, spinal stenosis, tumor, or rarely, infection. Patients suffering from lumbar myelopathy or cauda equina syndrome will experience varying degrees of lower extremity weakness and bowel and bladder symptomatology. This represents a neurosurgical emergency and should be treated as such.

TESTING

Magnetic resonance imaging of the lumbar spine will provide the clinician with the best information regarding the lumbar spine and its contents. MRI is highly accurate and will help identify abnormalities that may put the patient at risk for the development of lumbar myelopathy (see Figs. 12.8 and 12.9). In patients who

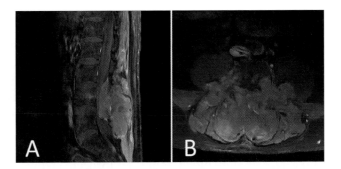

Fig. 12.9   Preoperative T1-weighted magnetic resonance image (MRI) with gadolinium administration. A sagittal image (A) demonstrates extent of paraspinal musculature involvement. An axial image (B) taken at the level of the L4 pedicles demonstrates near-complete spinal canal obliteration by the enhancing and expansile mass. (From Mehra RN, Ruan H, Park DH, Merkow MB, Chou D. Intradural osteogenic sarcoma in the lumbar spine. *J Clin Neurosci.* 2019;64:39−41, Fig. 1.)

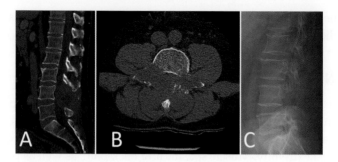

Fig. 12.10   Preoperative sagittal computed tomography (CT) (A) demonstrates absence of posterior elements at L4. Preoperative axial CT (B) at the level of the L4 pedicles and standing lumbar spine radiograph and (C) demonstrate complete lysis of the L4 pedicles. (From Mehra RN, Ruan H, Park DH, Merkow MB, Chou D. Intradural osteogenic sarcoma in the lumbar spine. *J Clin Neurosci.* 2019;64:39—41, Fig. 2.)

cannot undergo MRI (e.g., patients with a pacemaker), computed tomography or myelography is a reasonable second choice and may further elucidate bony abnormalities (Fig. 12.10). Discography may provide additional useful information in selected cases (Fig. 12.11). Radionuclide bone scanning and plain radiographs are indicated if fracture or bony abnormality, such as metastatic disease, is being considered. Although this testing provides the clinician with useful neuroanatomic information, electromyography and nerve conduction velocity testing will provide the clinician with neurophysiologic information that can delineate the actual status of each nerve root and the lumbar plexus. Screening laboratory testing consisting of complete blood count, erythrocyte sedimentation rate, and automated blood chemistry testing should be performed if the diagnosis of lumbar radiculopathy is in question.

DIFFERENTIAL DIAGNOSIS

Lumbar radiculopathy is a clinical diagnosis that is supported by a combination of clinical history, physical examination, radiography, and MRI. Pain syndromes that may mimic lumbar radiculopathy include low back strain, lumbar bursitis, lumbar fibromyositis, inflammatory arthritis, and disorders of the lumbar spinal cord, roots, plexus, and nerves (see Table 12.2). MRI of the lumbar spine should be carried out on all patients suspected of suffering from lumbar radiculopathy. Screening laboratory testing consisting of complete blood count, erythrocyte sedimentation rate, antinuclear antibody testing, HLA-B27 antigen screening, and automated blood chemistry testing should be performed if the diagnosis of lumbar radiculopathy is in question to help rule out other causes of the patient's pain.

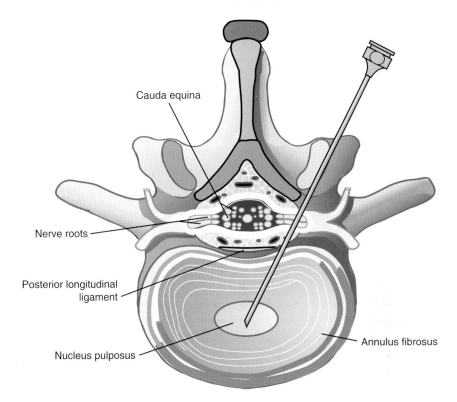

Fig. 12.11 Technique for lumbar discography. (From Waldman SD. *Atlas of Interventional Pain Management*. 4th ed. Philadelphia: Saunders; 2015: Fig. 150.6.)

THE INTERVERTEBRAL DISC

The lumbar intervertebral disc has two major functions. The first is to serve as the major shock-absorbing structure of the lumbar spine, and the second is to facilitate the synchronized movement of the lumbar spine while helping to prevent impingement of the neural structures and vasculature that traverse the lumbar spine. Both the shock-absorbing function and the movement/protective function of the lumbar intervertebral disc are functions of the disc structure, as well as of the laws of physics that affect it.

To understand how the lumbar intervertebral disc functions in health and becomes dysfunctional in disease, it is useful to think of the disc as a closed fluid-filled container. The outside of the container is made up of a top and bottom, called the endplates, which are composed of relatively inflexible hyaline cartilage. The sides of the lumbar intervertebral disc are made up of a woven criss-crossing matrix of fibroelastic fibers that tightly attaches to the top and bottom endplates (Fig. 12.12). This woven matrix of fibers is called the annulus, and it completely surrounds the sides of the disc. The interlaced structure of the

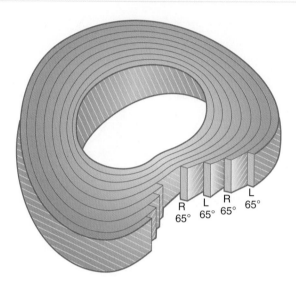

Fig. 12.12 The annulus surrounds the nucleus propulsus and is made up of collagen fibers arranged in multiple concentric layers with consecutive rings running in alternate directions. (From Waldman SD. *Atlas of Interventional Pain Management.* 4th ed. Philadelphia: Saunders; 2015: Fig. 12.13.)

annulus results in an enclosing mesh that is extremely strong, yet is very flexible, which facilitates the compression of the disc during the wide range of motion of the lumbar spine.

Inside this container consisting of the top and bottom endplates and surrounding annulus is the water-containing mucopolysaccharide gel-like substance called the nucleus pulposus (see Fig. 10.12A). The nucleus is incompressible and transmits any pressure placed on one portion of the disc to the surrounding nucleus. In health, the water-filled gel creates a positive intradiscal pressure, which forces apart the adjacent vertebra and helps protect the spinal cord and exiting nerve roots. When the lumbar spine moves, the incompressible nature of the nucleus pulposus maintains a constant intradiscal pressure while some fibers of the disc relax and others contract.

As the lumbar intervertebral disc ages, it becomes less vascular and loses its ability to absorb water into the disc (see Fig. 10.12B-D). This results in degradation of the disc's shock-absorbing and motion-facilitating functions. This problem worsens with degeneration of the annulus, which allows portions of the disc wall to bulge, distorting the ability of the nucleus pulposus to distribute evenly the forces placed on it throughout the entire disc. This exacerbates disc dysfunction and can contribute to further disc deterioration, which may ultimately lead to actual complete disruption of the annulus and extrusion of the nucleus. Intervertebral discs may herniate laterally, posteriorly, and anteriorly, as well as superiorly or inferiorly through weakened vertebral endplates. The deterioration of the disc is responsible for many of the painful conditions emanating from the lumbar spine that are encountered in clinical practice.

MANAGEMENT AND TREATMENT

Lumbar radiculopathy is best treated with a multimodality approach. Physical therapy, including heat modalities and deep sedative massage, combined with nonsteroidal antiinflammatory agents and skeletal muscle relaxants, represents a reasonable starting point. The addition of caudal or lumbar steroid epidural nerve blocks is a reasonable next step (Fig. 12.13). Caudal or lumbar epidural blocks with local anesthetic and steroids have been shown to be extremely effective in the treatment of lumbar radiculopathy. Underlying sleep disturbance and depression are best treated with a tricyclic antidepressant compound such as nortriptyline, which can be started at a single bedtime dose of 25 mg. If conservative therapy fails to relieve the patient's pain and neurologic symptoms, surgical management may be required.

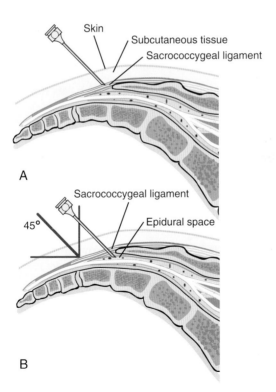

Fig. 12.13 Caudal epidural block. (A) Needle impinging on the sacrococcygeal ligament. (B) Needle passing through the sacrococcygeal ligament into the caudal epidural space. (From Waldman SD. *Atlas of Interventional Pain Management*. 4th ed. Philadelphia: Saunders; 2015: Fig. 105.9.)

HIGH-YIELD TAKEAWAYS

- The patient is afebrile, making an acute infectious etiology (e.g., epidural abscess) unlikely.
- The patient's symptomatology is the result of acute trauma to the lumbar intervertebral disc.
- The patient's pain is localized in the back and right lower extremity, which is highly suggestive of lumbar radiculopathy.
- The patient's symptoms are unilateral, which would be more suggestive of lumbar radiculopathy vs. other pathologic processes, although bilateral radiculopathy is not that uncommon.
- The patient's neurologic examination is abnormal in the affected right lower extremity with S1 sensory deficit, ankle everter weakness, and a diminished ankle jerk reflex, which is highly suggestive of a right S1 radiculopathy.
- There are no bowel or bladder symptoms or pathologic reflexes suggestive of myelopathy.
- MRI scanning is highly sensitive in the diagnosis of discogenic disease and is useful in ruling out other space-occupying lesions that may be producing radicular symptoms.

Suggested Readings

Barr K. Electrodiagnosis of lumbar radiculopathy. *Phys Med Rehabil Clin N Am.* 2013:24 (1):79−91.

Waldman SD. Functional anatomy of the lumbar spine. In: *Physical Diagnosis of Pain: An Atlas of Signs and Symptoms.* 4th ed. Philadelphia: Elsevier; 2020.

Waldman SD. Lumbar epidural nerve block: Interlaminar approach. In: *Atlas of Interventional Pain Management.* 4th ed. Philadelphia: Elsevier; 2015:500−513.

Waldman SD. Lumbar radiculopathy. In: *Pain Review.* 2nd ed. Philadelphia: Saunders; 2017:256−257.

Waldman SD. The Lesegue straight leg raiding test for lumbar radiculopathy. In: *Physical Diagnosis of Pain: An Atlas of Signs and Symptoms.* 3rd ed. Philadelphia: Elsevier; 2016:235−236.

Waldman SD, Campbell RSD. Anatomy: Special imaging considerations of the lumbar spine. In: *Imaging of Pain.* Philadelphia: Elsevier; 2011:109−110.

Carmen Delarosa

A 26-Year-Old Female With
Back Pain and Bilateral Lower
Extremity Weakness

LEARNING OBJECTIVES

- Learn the common causes of low back pain and lumbar radiculopathy.
- Develop an understanding of the role of the lumbar instability in low back pain.
- Develop an understanding of the causes of lumbar instability.
- Learn the clinical presentation of lumbar instability.
- Learn how to use physical examination to determine which lumbar spinal nerve roots are subserving the patient's pain.
- Learn to distinguish lumbar strain from lumbar radiculopathy.
- Learn the important anatomic structures involved in lumbar instability.
- Develop an understanding of the treatment options for lumbar instability.
- Learn the appropriate testing options to help diagnose low back pain and lumbar instability.
- Learn to identify red flags waving in patients who present with lumbar instability.

Carmen Delarosa

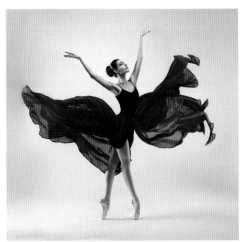

Carmen Delarosa is a 26-year-old ballet dancer with the chief complaint of, "I missed a *sissonne* and I felt something give in my back and now my legs are getting weak." She noted that before the accident, "My back had been bothering me off and on for the last 7 or 8 months. As you know, Doctor, back pain is kind of an occupational hazard for dancers. In the past, when my back played up, I would do my stretching exercises and use a heating pad and it would always get better...but this time it is different...I can't seem to get better."

"What about Tylenol, Motrin, pain pills?" I asked. "Oh no, doctor, I don't believe in putting any of that poison in my body...only natural things and clean foods." I asked, "OK, so are there any other symptoms associated with your back pain...numbness, tingling, arm or leg weakness...anything else?" Carmen answered, "Not really, Doctor...but sometimes it feels like the top of my right foot has gone to sleep or something...not all the time, just sometimes...especially when I have been standing for a long time. Doctor, I know this may sound crazy, but sometimes, when I go for a walk around the block to try and keep from going stir crazy...after I walk for a while...it feels like my legs are getting weak. I know that it's probably just my imagination." "Ms. Delarosa, are you having any difficulty when you go to the bathroom...losing any urine, having accidents?" Carmen said, "No, not really...but it really hurts to get up from the commode."

Carmen's physical examination was not all that remarkable. She was really fit. Her head, ears, eyes, nose, and throat (HEENT), cardiopulmonary, and abdominal examinations were completely normal. She had a resting pulse of 58 and was normotensive and afebrile. Her neck examination was normal, as was her upper extremity neurologic examination. I thought that her dorsiflexors on the right lower extremity might be just a little weak, but I couldn't be sure. Despite Carmen's report of a pins and needles sensation across the top of the right foot, I couldn't really identify any clear sensory deficits in either leg. Deep tendon reflexes were physiologic bilaterally. There were no pathologic reflexes or clonus.

Examination of her back revealed significant pain on flexion, extension, and lateral bending. I asked Carmen to continue standing and to face the examination table, then place the palms of her hands flat on the edge of the table. I then asked her to walk backward a few steps and then bow out her lumbar spine. I palpated each interspinous space to evaluate the relative positions of the upper spinous processes to the adjacent lower spinous processes. I was looking for a wider than normal interspinous gap, which would suggest lumbar spine instability. I then asked Carmen to keep her feet in the same position and push her pelvis toward the examination table to extend her lumbar spine. I repalpated each interspinous space and it felt like there was an increased interspinous gap at the L5-S1 interspace. I was beginning to get the picture.

Key Clinical Points—What's Important and What's Not

THE HISTORY

- A history of acute trauma from a dancing injury
- A history of previous intermittent back pain
- Sensation that the legs get weak after walking some distance
- Intermittent pins and needles sensation across the dorsum of the right foot
- No bowel or bladder symptomatology

THE PHYSICAL EXAMINATION

- The patient is afebrile
- Normal sensory examination despite a subjective complaint of an intermittent pins and needles sensation across the dorsum of the right foot
- Decreased sensation down the back of the leg and into the dorsum of the foot (Fig. 13.1)
- Questionable weakness of the extensor hallucis longus on the right (Fig. 13.2)
- Positive interspinous gap test (Fig. 13.3)
- Normal left upper extremity motor and sensory examination
- No pathologic reflexes
- No clonus
- Positive Lasegue sign bilaterally (Fig. 13.4)

OTHER FINDINGS OF NOTE

- Normal HEENT examination
- Normal cardiovascular examination
- Normal pulmonary examination
- Normal abdominal examination
- No peripheral edema

SENSORY

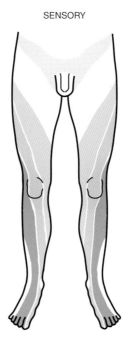

Fig. 13.1 Sensory distribution of the L5 dermatome (turquoise). (From Waldman SD. *Physical Diagnosis of Pain: An Atlas of Signs and Symptoms*. 3rd ed. St. Louis: Elsevier; 2020: Fig 145.1.)

MOTOR

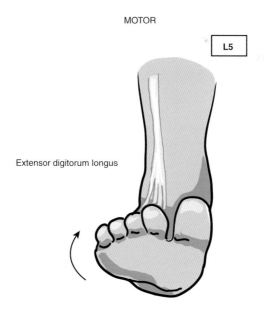

Fig. 13.2 L5 manual muscle testing. (From Waldman SD. *Physical Diagnosis of Pain: An Atlas of Signs and Symptoms*. 3rd ed. St. Louis: Elsevier; 2020: Fig 145.2.)

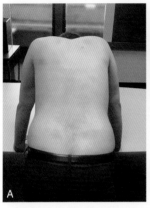
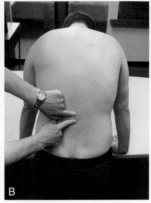
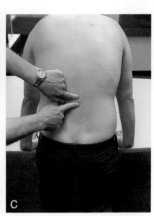

Fig. 13.3 Interspinous gap test. (A) Patients are asked to place their feet at shoulder width, place their palms flat on the examination table, and take three steps back to flex the lumbar spine. (B) With the patient's spine flexed, the examiner palpates each interspinous gap to identify asymmetry and abnormal widening. (C) Patients are then asked to thrust their pelvis toward the examination table to extend the lumbar spine. The examiner again palpates each interspinous gap to identify asymmetry and abnormal widening. (Courtesy Steven Waldman, MD.)

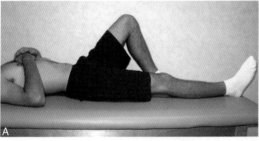
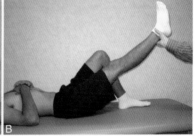

Fig. 13.4 Lasegue sign testing. The Lasegue straight leg raising test. (A) The patient is in the supine position with the unaffected leg flexed to 45 degrees at the knee and the affected leg placed flat against the table. (B) With the ankle of the affected leg placed at 90 degrees of flexion, the affected leg is slowly raised toward the ceiling while the knee is kept fully extended. (From Waldman SD. *Physical Diagnosis of Pain: An Atlas of Signs and Symptoms*. 3rd ed. St. Louis: Elsevier; 2020: Fig 147.1 and 147.2.)

What Tests Would You Like To Order?

The following tests were ordered:
- Plain radiograph of the lumbar spine
- Magnetic resonance image (MRI) scan of the lumbar spine
- Electromyography and nerve conduction testing of the back and the right lower extremity.

TEST RESULTS

- The plain radiographs revealed a type 2a isthmic spondylolisthesis. Lateral radiograph of the lumbar spine demonstrates bilateral L4 pars defects (*arrow*) with associated grade 1 L4/5 isthmic spondylolisthesis. The L4/5 disc had degeneration (Fig. 13.5).
- The MRI revealed a grade 2 spondylolisthesis of L4 on L5 (Fig. 13.6). Electromyography and nerve conduction testing reveals findings consistent with an L5-S1 radiculopathy.

 Clinical Correlation—Putting It All Together

What is the diagnosis?
- Spondylolisthesis L5 on S1 with possible pseudoclaudication

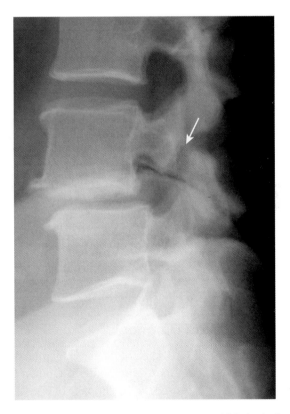

Fig. 13.5 Plain radiograph demonstrating a type 2a isthmic spondylolisthesis. Lateral radiograph of the lumbar spine demonstrates bilateral L4 pars defects (*arrow*) with associated grade 1 L4/5 isthmic spondylolisthesis. The L4/5 disc has degeneration. (From Waldman S: *Atlas of Uncommon Pain Syndromes*. 3rd ed. Philadelphia, Saunders; 2014: Fig 78.2.)

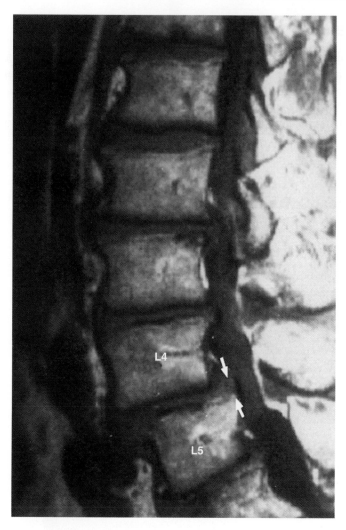

Fig. 13.6 Magnetic resonance image (MRI) of the lumbar spine revealing a grade 2 spondylolisthesis of L4 on L5. This leads to the false impression of L4-5 disc herniation. (From Waldman SD. *Atlas of Uncommon Pain Syndromes*. 3rd ed. Philadelphia: Saunders; 2014: Fig 78.3.)

The Science Behind the Diagnosis

Spondylolisthesis is a degenerative disease of the lumbar spine that results in pain and functional disability. It occurs more commonly in women and is most often seen after age 40. This disease is caused by the slippage of one vertebral body onto another. Usually, the upper vertebral body moves anteriorly relative to the vertebral body below it, which causes narrowing of the spinal canal. This narrowing creates a relative spinal stenosis and back pain and if sufficiently severe, can lead to cauda equina syndrome. Occasionally, the upper vertebral body slides

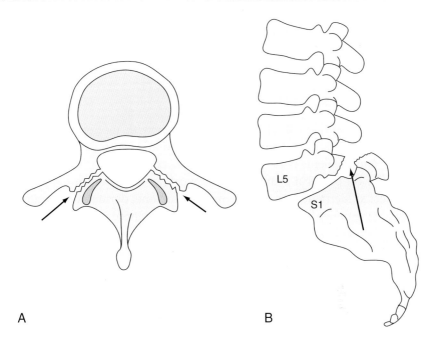

A   B

Fig. 13.7 (A) Spondylolysis with bilateral defects in the pars interarticularis (*arrows*). (B) Spondylolysis of the L5 vertebra (*arrow*) resulting in isthmic spondylolisthesis at L5-S1. (From Firestein G, Budd R, Gabriel SE, McInnes IB, O'Dell J. *Kelley and Firestein's Textbook of Rheumatology*. 10th ed. Philadelphia: Elsevier; 2017: Fig. 47.7.)

TABLE 13.1 ■ **Classification of Spondylolisthesis**

Type	Pathology
Dysplastic	Congenital dysplasia of articular processes
Isthmic	Pars articularis defect
Degenerative	Facet joint degeneration
Traumatic	Neural arch fracture other than pars interarticularis
Pathologic	Neural arch failure secondary to bone disease
Iatrogenic	Excessive surgical bone removal during spine surgery

posteriorly relative to the vertebral body below it, which compromises the neural foramina. This is known as retrolisthesis. There are several types of spondylolisthesis and a classification system has been developed to help classify the pathology responsible for the vertebral instability (Fig. 13.7, Table 13.1).

SPONDYLOLISTHESIS

Clinically, a patient with spondylolisthesis reports back pain with lifting, twisting, or bending of the lumbar spine. Patients may state that they feel like they have "a catch in their back." Patients with spondylolisthesis often report radicular pain of the lower extremity and often experience pseudoclaudication with walking. Rarely, the slippage of the vertebra is so extreme that myelopathy or cauda equina syndrome develops.

SIGNS AND SYMPTOMS

Patients with spondylolisthesis report back pain with motion of the lumbar spine. Rising from a sitting to a standing position often reproduces the pain (Fig. 13.8). Many patients with spondylolisthesis experience radicular symptoms that manifest on physical examination as weakness and sensory abnormality in the affected dermatomes. Often, more than one dermatome is affected. Occasionally, a patient with spondylolisthesis experiences compression of the lumbar spinal nerve roots and cauda equina, resulting in myelopathy or cauda equina syndrome. Lumbar myelopathy is most commonly caused by a midline herniated lumbar disc, spinal stenosis, tumor, or rarely, infection. Patients with lumbar myelopathy or cauda equina syndrome experience varying degrees of

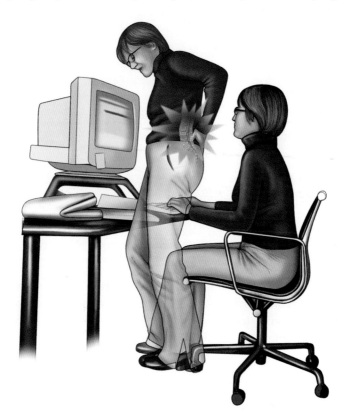

Fig. 13.8 Patients with spondylolisthesis often report back pain with motion of the lumbar spine. Rising from a sitting to a standing position often reproduces the pain. (From Waldman SD. *Atlas of Uncommon Pain Syndromes*. 3rd ed. Philadelphia: Saunders; 2014: Fig 78.1.)

lower extremity weakness and bowel and bladder symptoms; this represents a neurosurgical emergency and should be treated as such.

TESTING

Plain radiographs of the lumbar spine usually are sufficient to diagnose spondylolisthesis (see Fig. 13.5). The lateral view shows the slippage of one vertebra onto another. MRI of the lumbar spine provides the best information regarding the contents of the lumbar spine (see Figs. 13.6, 13.9, 13.10). MRI is highly accurate and helps identify abnormalities that may put the patient at risk for the development of lumbar myelopathy, such as the trefoil spinal canal of congenital spinal stenosis and other causes of low back pain and radiculopathy (Fig. 13.11). In patients who cannot undergo MRI, such as patients with pacemakers, computed tomography (CT) and myelography are reasonable second choices (Fig. 13.12). Radionucleotide bone scanning and plain radiographs are indicated if fracture or bony abnormality, such as metastatic disease, is being considered.

Although imaging provides useful neuroanatomic information, electromyography and nerve conduction velocity testing provide neurophysiologic information that can delineate the actual status of each nerve root and the lumbar plexus. Screening laboratory tests consisting of complete blood cell count, erythrocyte

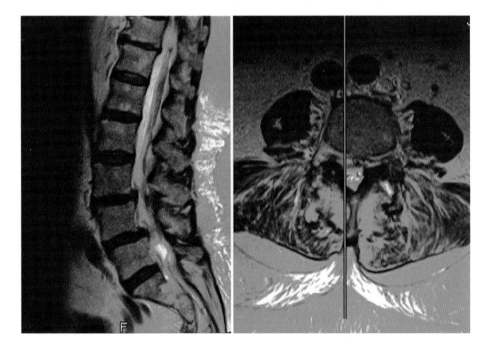

Fig. 13.9 Magnetic resonance image (MRI) of the lumbar spine demonstrating significant spondylosis and spondylolisthesis. (From Yue J, Guyer R, Johnson JP, Khoo L, Hochschuler S. *The Comprehensive Treatment of the Aging Spine*. Philadelphia: Saunders; 2011: Fig. 13.1.)

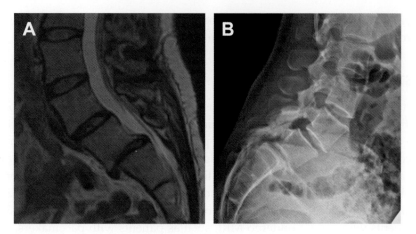

Fig. 13.10   (A) Sagittal T2-weighted magnetic resonance image (MRI). With incompetence of the posterior elements from defects in the pars interarticularis, the intervertebral disc is subject to shearing stress, resulting in further disc degeneration and translation of the cephalad on caudal vertebrae. (B) Lateral radiograph demonstrating a grade 2 isthmic spondylolisthesis with at least 25%, but less than 50% translation of L5 on S1. (From: Bhalla A, Bono C. Isthmic lumbar spondylolisthesis. *Neurosurg Clin N Am*. 2019;30(3):283−290, Fig. 1.)

sedimentation rate, and automated blood chemistry testing should be performed if the diagnosis of spondylolisthesis is in question.

DIFFERENTIAL DIAGNOSIS

Spondylolisthesis is a radiographic diagnosis that is supported by a combination of clinical history, physical examination, radiography, and MRI. Pain syndromes that may mimic spondylolisthesis include lumbar radiculopathy, low back strain, lumbar bursitis, lumbar fibromyositis, inflammatory arthritis, and disorders of the lumbar spinal cord, roots, plexus, and nerves. MRI of the lumbar spine should be performed in all patients thought to have spondylolisthesis not only to clarify the type of spondylolisthesis responsible for the patient's pain and neurologic dysfunction but also to identify other potentially treatable pathology contributing to the patient's symptoms (Fig. 13.13). Screening laboratory tests consisting of complete blood cell count, erythrocyte sedimentation rate, antinuclear antibody testing, human leukocyte antigen (HLA) B-27 antigen screening, and automated blood chemistry testing should be performed if the diagnosis of spondylolisthesis is in question to help rule out other causes of pain.

TREATMENT

Spondylolisthesis is best treated with a multimodality approach. Physical therapy, including flexion exercises, heat modalities, and deep sedative massage,

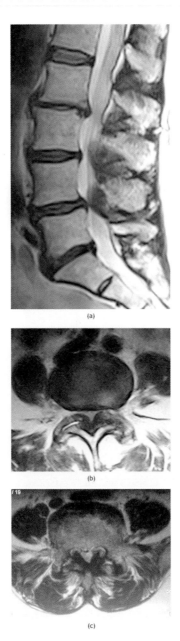

(a)

(b)

(c)

Fig. 13.11 Degenerative spondylolisthesis and associated spinal stenosis. (A) Sagittal T2-weighted fast spin echo (FSE) magnetic resonance image (MRI) shows L4/5 spondylolisthesis and central canal stenosis, manifest as complete loss of cerebrospinal fluid around the cauda equina. (B) Axial T2-weighted FSE MRI through the L4/5 disc shows severe central canal stenosis and marked thickening of the ligamentum flavum. (C) Axial T2-weighted FSE MRI at the L5 pedicle level shows compression of both L5 roots within the lateral recesses owing to the forward slip of the inferior articular processes. (From Butt S, Saifuddin A. The imaging of lumbar spondylolisthesis. *Clin Radiol.* 2005;60(5):533–546, Fig. 11.)

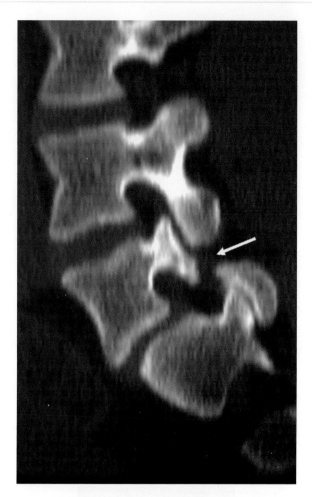

Fig. 13.12 Computed tomography demonstrating pars defect. A sagittal oblique multiplanar reconstruction demonstrates a pars interarticularis defect at L4 (*arrow*) with a few millimeters of spondylolisthesis of L4 on L5 (grade 1). (From Waldman SD, Bloch *J. Pain Management*. 2e, Philadelphia:
Saunders; 2007: Fig. 9.9.)

combined with nonsteroidal antiinflammatory drugs and skeletal muscle relaxants, represents a reasonable starting point. The addition of steroid epidural
nerve blocks is a reasonable next step. Caudal or lumbar epidural blocks with a
local anesthetic and steroid have been shown to be extremely effective in the
treatment of pain secondary to spondylolisthesis. Underlying sleep disturbance
and depression are best treated with a tricyclic antidepressant compound, such
as nortriptyline, which can be started at a single bedtime dose of 25 mg. In
patients who fail to respond to conservative treatment or have significant or progressive neurologic symptoms, surgical fixation of the vertebral instability may
be required (Fig. 13.14).

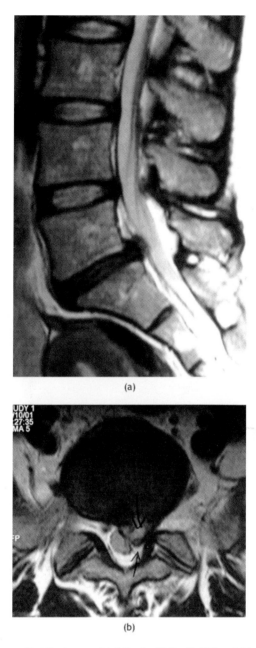

(a)

(b)

Fig. 13.13 Disc prolapse with isthmic spondylolisthesis. (A) Sagittal T2-weighted fast spin echo (FSE) magnetic resonance image (MRI) shows L5/S1 isthmic spondylolisthesis with associated disc prolapse. Note the increased anteroposterior canal dimension, which differentiates isthmic spondylolisthesis from degenerative spondylolisthesis. (B) Axial T2-weighted FSE MRI shows a left paracentral L5/S1 disc prolapse with compression of the left S1 nerve root. (From Butt S, Saifuddin A. The imaging of lumbar spondylolisthesis. *Clin Radiol*. 2005;(5):533–546, Fig. 8.)

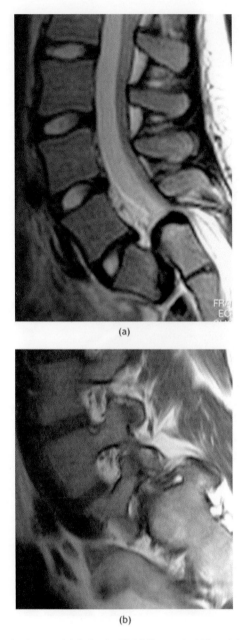

(a)

(b)

Fig. 13.14 Type 1a dysplastic spondylolisthesis. (A) Midline sagittal T2-weighted fast spin echo (FSE) magnetic resonance image (MRI) demonstrates a degenerate pseudobulging lumbosacral disc with severe compression of the cauda equina between the neural arch of L4 and the superoposterior aspect of the sacrum. (B) Parasagittal T1-weighted SE MRI at the level of the intervertebral foramen shows severe compression of the exiting L5 nerve root. (From Butt S, Saifuddin A. The imaging of lumbar spondylolisthesis. *Clin Radiol.* 2005;(5):533–546, Fig. 3.)

HIGH-YIELD TAKEAWAYS

- The patient is afebrile, making an acute infectious etiology (e.g., epidural abscess) unlikely.
- The patient's symptomatology is the result of acute trauma secondary to a dance injury.
- The patient's pain is localized in the back and with some right lower extremity symptoms.
- The patient's neurologic symptoms are unilateral, which would be more suggestive of lumbar radiculopathy vs. other pathologic processes, although bilateral radiculopathy is not that uncommon.
- The patient has significant pain with range of motion of the lumbar spine.
- The interspinous gap examination is abnormal, which is suggestive of lumbar instability.
- The neurologic examination is not significantly abnormal.
- There are no bowel or bladder symptoms or pathologic reflexes suggestive of myelopathy or cauda equina syndrome.
- There are multiple causes of spondylolisthesis.
- MRI scanning is highly sensitive in the diagnosis of discogenic disease and is useful in ruling out other space-occupying lesions that may be producing the patient's symptoms (see Figs. 13.13 and 13.14).

Suggested Readings

Waldman SD. Spondylolisthesis. In: *Atlas of Uncommon Pain Syndromes*. 3rd ed. Philadelphia: Saunders; 2014:227—229.

Waldman SD. Functional anatomy of the lumbar spine. In: *Physical Diagnosis of Pain: An Atlas of Signs and Symptoms*. 4th ed. Philadelphia: Elsevier; 2020:237—238.

Xiáng Y, Wáng J, Wu A-M, Santiago FR, Nogueira-Barbosa MH. Informed appropriate imaging for low back pain management: a narrative review. *J Orthop Transl*. 2018;15:21—34. 2018.

Barr K. Electrodiagnosis of lumbar radiculopathy. *Phys Med Rehabil Clin North Am*. 2013;24(1):79—91.

Waldman SD. Lumbar epidural nerve block: interlaminar approach. *Atlas of Interventional Pain Management*. 4th ed. Philadelphia: Elsevier; 2015:500—513.

Waldman SD. The Lesegue straight leg raising test for lumbar radiculopathy. In: *Physical Diagnosis of Pain: An Atlas of Signs and Symptoms*. 3rd ed. Philadelphia: Elsevier; 2016:235—236.

Waldman SD, Campbell RSD. Anatomy: Special imaging considerations of the lumbar spine. In: *Imaging of Pain*. Philadelphia: Elsevier; 2011:109—110.

Declan Mulroney

A 48-Year-Old Male With Lower Extremity Cramping and Weakness With Ambulation

- Learn the common causes of lower extremity pain and weakness when walking.
- Learn the clinical presentation of spinal stenosis.
- Learn to distinguish spinal stenosis from vascular insufficiency of the lower extremities.
- Learn the anatomic structures involved in the evolution of spinal stenosis.
- Develop an understanding of the treatment options for spinal stenosis.
- Develop an understanding of other painful conditions that may mimic spinal stenosis.
- Develop an understanding of the role of interventional pain management in the treatment of lumbar strain.

Declan Mulroney

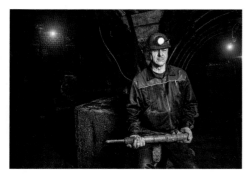

Declan Mulroney is a 48-year-old miner with a chief complaint of, "My legs cramp up and get weak when I walk for any distance." Declan noted that over the last six months, he had been having trouble walking any distance at all. When he walked, his legs start to cramp and then they feel like they are going to give out.

Declan went on to say, "Whenever there is a safety issue, it's my job to get everybody topside ASAP until I can sort things out and make sure it's safe to go back to work. So, I count heads to make sure I've got everybody and herd everybody out...everybody was pretty worked up, so we were walking pretty fast. It was a pretty long walk to get topside...about a mile...and I was walking behind the guys to keep them moving. So, we got about halfway out and my legs started cramping up. But the rules are the rules, and I needed to get everybody topside ASAP, so I just kept pushing on, even though my legs were really cramping up...and then...my legs started getting weak."

"I don't think any of the guys figured it out...but Doctor, this keeps happening...and I feel like over the last few months, it's been getting worse. If my legs give out at the wrong time, I could get me and my crew killed." Declan dropped his head and looked back down at the floor and said, "Doctor, I went on the Internet to try and figure out what was wrong with my legs...and..." Declan stopped and took a deep breath...he then raised his head and looked me straight in the eye. He took a couple more big breaths and in a shaky, but determined voice, he asked..."Doctor...do you think I have Lou Gehrig's disease?"

"Declan, I'm going to ask you a lot of questions that should help point us in the right direction." "Fine Doctor, fire away," Declan responded. "So, Declan, I understand that you are having leg cramping with walking and if you keep walking after the cramping starts, you feel like your legs are going to give out. Is that correct?" "That's right," he said. "Do you have any numbness or pain in your legs right now as we are talking?" Declan shook his head. "Any weight loss, fever, chills, difficulty swallowing, feeling poorly," I asked? "Absolutely not," Declan said emphatically, "you know I'm strong as a horse." "So," I said, "I know that after you walk for a while, your legs feel like they are going to give out...do you have anything like that in your arms...are you dropping things...do your arms feel weak...do you feel clumsy?" "Doc," Declan said, "My arms and hands are fine...it's my legs I'm worried about." "I understand...are you having any problem peeing or pooping...having any accidents or anything like that?" "No Doc, I'm as regular as a clock."

"Declan, is there anything that makes the cramping and feeling of fatigue worse...anything that makes it better?" I asked? A thoughtful look spread across Declan's face as he said, "Funny you should ask that. Whenever I am looking up to inspect the back..." he laughed and said..."You know...the roof—...if I look up for very long, I start getting that cramping feeling in both of my legs. If I look back down and sort of bend my knees and bend my back forward a little...after a minute or two, the pain goes away."

I asked Declan to walk for me. So he got off the examination table and walked down the hall. I watched Declan walk to the end of the hallway and back. After a couple of trips back and forth, I noticed that Declan was slowing down and was starting to assume a simian posture. I asked, "Hey Declan, are you starting to have the cramping in your legs?" He kept walking and with an amazed look, said, "Yes, how did you know?" "Let's get you back on the examination table and wind this up." "You got it, Doc...I'm about walked out," Declan responded as he headed back to the examination room.

On physical examination, Declan was afebrile and normotensive. His head, ears, eyes, nose, and throat (HEENT) examination, including a careful fundoscopic examination, was completely normal, as was his cardiopulmonary examination. I had him stick out his tongue and there were no fasciculations there, nor were there any in the interosseous muscles of his hands. I really didn't think he had amyotropic lateral sclerosis...but you never know. His abdominal examination was normal. There was no abnormal mass or organomegaly, nor was there peripheral edema. Declan's neurologic examination was normal. Specifically, his upper and lower extremity deep tendon reflexes were physiologic and there was no sensory deficit or weakness. There was no clonus and I could not elicit any pathologic reflexes. There were no trophic skin changes on his feet or toes, and the hair growth on his distal lower extremities was normal. Dorsalis pedis and posterior tibialis pulses were full. There was no costovertebral angle tenderness, nor was there tenderness to palpation of the paraspinous muscles. The Lasegue test was negative bilaterally. I decided to perform a stoop test. I had Declan sit up as straight as he could for two minutes and asked if he was feeling any cramping in his legs...and as expected, the answer was yes (Fig. 14.1). I then asked him to flex his lower back forward and tell me what was going on with his pain. After about thirty seconds, he said the pain was completely gone.

I checked to see that Declan was up to date on his immunizations, which he was. I then told him that I was pretty sure that he didn't have Lou Gehrig's disease, but we would get a few tests just to be sure.

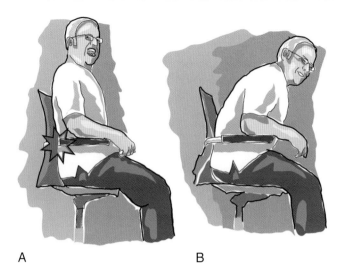

A   B

Fig. 14.1   Stoop test for spinal stenosis. (A) Extension of the lumbar spine exacerbates the pain of spinal stenosis. (B) Flexion of the lumbar spine relieves the pain of spinal stenosis. (From Waldman SD. *Atlas of Common Pain Syndromes*. 4th ed. Philadelphia: Elsevier; 2019: Fig. 84.4.)

Key Clinical Points—What's Important and What's Not

THE HISTORY

- Chief complaint of "lower extremity cramping and feeling like my legs are going to give out"
- Onset of symptoms came on gradually over time
- No history of acute trauma
- Lack of significant antecedent trauma to back (e.g., motor vehicle accident, fall)
- Inability to stand up straight
- No clear pain radiation into lower extremities
- No numbness of lower extremities unless walking for a moderate distance
- Symptoms triggered by extension of the lumbar spine
- Symptoms relieved by flexion of the lumbar spine
- No urinary or fecal incontinence
- No pathologic reflexes

THE PHYSICAL EXAMINATION

- The patient is afebrile
- Patient assumes simian posture after walking for a moderate distance
- No fasciculations of the tongue or fine muscles of the hand
- Positive stoop test (see Fig. 14.1)
- Normal deep tendon reflexes

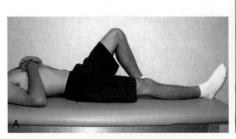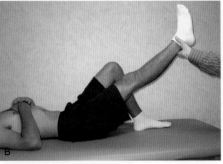

Fig. 14.2 The Lasègue straight leg raising test. (A) With the patient in the supine position, the unaffected leg is flexed 45 degrees at the knee, and the affected leg is placed flat against the table. (B) With the ankle of the affected leg placed at 90 degrees of flexion, the affected leg is slowly raised toward the ceiling while the knee is kept fully extended. (From Waldman SD. *Atlas of Common Pain Syndromes*. 4th ed. Philadelphia: Elsevier; 2019: Fig. 82.2.)

- Normal upper and lower extremity motor and sensory examination
- No evidence of vascular insufficiency
- No pathologic reflexes
- No clonus
- Negative Lasegue sign (Fig. 14.2)

OTHER FINDINGS OF NOTE

- Normal cardiovascular examination
- Normal pulmonary examination
- Normal abdominal examination
- No peripheral edema

 What Tests Would You Like to Order?

The following tests were ordered:
- Magnetic resonance imaging (MRI) of the lumbar spine
- Electromyography and nerve conduction velocity testing of the lower extremities bilaterally
- Doppler vascular studies of the lower extremities to rule out vascular claudication

TEST RESULTS

The MRI scan of Declan's lumbar spine revealed significant degenerative spinal stenosis with a decreased anteroposterior diameter of the neural canal at the L4-L5 level owing to redundancy of the ligamentum flavum, complicated by

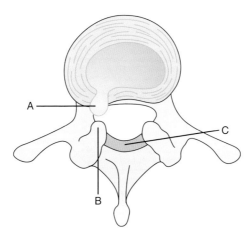

Fig. 14.3 Degenerative spinal stenosis. (A) The sagittal T2-weighted magnetic resonance image shows decreased anteroposterior diameter of the neural canal at the L4-L5 level owing to redundancy of the ligamentum flavum. (B) The axial image through the L4-L5 disc shows decreased cross-sectional area of the thecal sac from hypertrophic changes of the facet joints posterolateral to the thecal sac. (C) Hypertrophy of ligamentum flavum. (From Firestein G, Budd RC, Gabriel SE, McInnes IB, O'Dell JR, Koretzky G. *Kelley and Firestein's Textbook of Rheumatology*. 10th ed. Philadelphia: Elsevier; 2017: Fig. 47.8.)

hypertrophic changes of the facet joints (Fig. 14.3). His electromyogram revealed a mild L5 radiculopathy bilaterally. Declan's nerve conduction velocity testing was normal. Doppler vascular flow studies of the bilateral lower extremities were reported as within normal limits for age.

 Clinical Correlation—Putting It All Together

What is the diagnosis?
- Spinal stenosis

The Science Behind the Diagnosis

Spinal stenosis is the result of congenital or acquired narrowing of the spinal canal. It occurs most commonly at the L5 vertebral level, with women affected more commonly than men. Clinically, spinal stenosis usually manifests in a characteristic manner as pain and weakness in the legs when walking. This neurogenic pain is called pseudoclaudication or neurogenic claudication (Fig. 14.4). These symptoms are usually accompanied by lower extremity pain emanating from the lumbar nerve roots. In addition, patients with spinal stenosis may experience numbness, weakness, and loss of reflexes. The causes of spinal stenosis include a bulging or herniated disc, facet arthropathy, and thickening and buckling of the

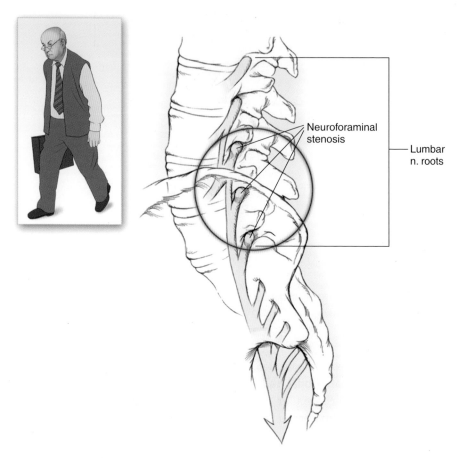

Fig. 14.4 Pseudoclaudication is the sine qua non of spinal stenosis. (From Waldman SD. *Atlas of Common Pain Syndromes*. 4th ed. Philadelphia: Saunders; 2019: Fig. 84.2.)

interlaminar ligaments (Box 14.1). All these inciting factors tend to worsen with age.

SIGNS AND SYMPTOMS

Patients suffering from spinal stenosis complain of calf and leg pain and fatigue when walking, standing, or lying supine. These symptoms disappear if they flex the lumbar spine or assume the sitting position. Frequently, patients suffering from spinal stenosis exhibit a simian posture, with a forward-flexed trunk and slightly bent knees when walking, to decrease the symptoms of pseudoclaudication (Fig. 14.5). Extension of the spine may cause an increase in symptoms. Patients also complain of pain, numbness, tingling, and paresthesias in the distribution of the affected nerve root or roots. Weakness and lack of coordination in

BOX 14.1 ■ Causes of Lumbar Spinal Stenosis

Congenital
- Idiopathic
- Achondroplastic

Acquired
Degenerative
- Spondylosis
- Spondylolisthesis
- Disc degeneration
- Disc herniation
- Hypertrophy of facet joints
- Hypertrophy of ligamentum flavum
- Scoliosis

Traumatic
Iatrogenic
- Postlaminectomy
- Postsurgical fusion
- Postsurgical perineural fibrosis
- Postmyelogram arachnoiditis

Infectious
- Discitis
- Paraspinal tubercular abscess
- Osteomyelitis

Rheumatic/Miscellaneous
- Miscellaneous space-occupying lesions
- Ankylosing spondylitis
- Rheumatoid arthritis
- Fluoride deposition

Metabolic
- Paget disease
- Acromegaly
- Diffuse idiopathic skeletal hyperostosis
- Hyperparathroidism
- Diffuse idiopathic hyperostosis
- Epidural lipomatosis
- X-linked hypophosphatemic osteomalacia

the affected extremity may be noted. Patients often have a positive stoop test for spinal stenosis (see Fig. 14.1). Muscle spasms and back pain, as well as pain referred to the trapezius and interscapular region, are common. Decreased sensation, weakness, and reflex changes are demonstrated on physical examination.

Occasionally, patients suffering from spinal stenosis experience compression of the lumbar spinal nerve roots and cauda equina, with resulting lumbar

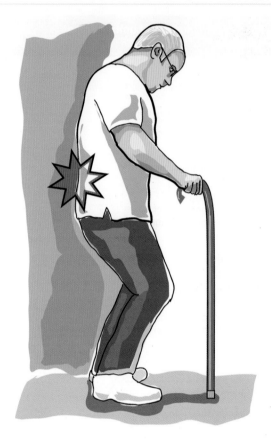

Fig. 14.5 Patients suffering from spinal stenosis often assume a simian posture, with a forward-flexed trunk and slightly bent knees when walking, to decrease the symptoms of pseudoclaudication. (From Waldman SD. *Physical Diagnosis of Pain: An Atlas of Signs and Symptoms*. Philadelphia: Saunders; 2006:260.)

myelopathy or cauda equina syndrome. These patients experience varying degrees of lower extremity weakness and bowel and bladder symptoms. This condition represents a neurosurgical emergency and should be treated as such, although the onset of symptoms is often insidious.

TESTING

Magnetic resonance imaging provides the best information about the lumbar spine and its contents and should be performed in all patients suspected of having spinal stenosis. MRI is highly accurate and can identify abnormalities that may put the patient at risk for lumbar myelopathy (Figs. 14.6 and 14.7). In patients who cannot undergo MRI (e.g., those with pacemakers), computed tomography (CT) or myelography is a reasonable alternative (Figs. 14.8 and 14.9). Radionuclide bone scanning and plain radiography are indicated if a

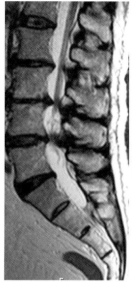
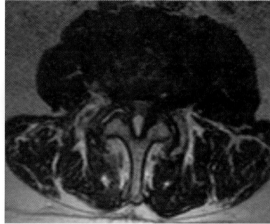

Fig. 14.6 Sagittal and axial T2-weighted images of a lumbar spinal stenosis patient, showing cerebrospinal fluid effacement caused by both anterior and posterior compression. In the axial image (on the *right*) facet hypertrophy leading to foraminal stenosis can be noted. (From Biller J, Ferro J. *Handbook of Clinical Neurology*, Vol. 119. Amsterdam: Elsevier; 2014: Fig. 35.3.)

coexistent fracture or bony abnormality, such as metastatic disease, is being considered.

Although MRI, CT, and myelography can supply useful neuroanatomic information, electromyography and nerve conduction velocity testing provide neurophysiologic information about the actual status of each nerve root and the lumbar plexus. Electromyography can also distinguish plexopathy from radiculopathy and can identify a coexistent entrapment neuropathy that may confuse the diagnosis.

If the diagnosis is in question, laboratory tests consisting of a complete blood count, erythrocyte sedimentation rate, antinuclear antibody testing, human leukocyte antigen (HLA)-B27 screening, and automated blood chemistry should be performed to rule out other causes of the patient's pain.

DIFFERENTIAL DIAGNOSIS

Spinal stenosis is a clinical diagnosis supported by a combination of clinical history, physical examination, radiography, and MRI. Pain syndromes that may mimic spinal stenosis include low back strain; lumbar bursitis; lumbar fibromyositis; inflammatory arthritis; and disorders of the lumbar spinal cord, roots, plexus, and nerves, including diabetic femoral neuropathy (Box 14.2).

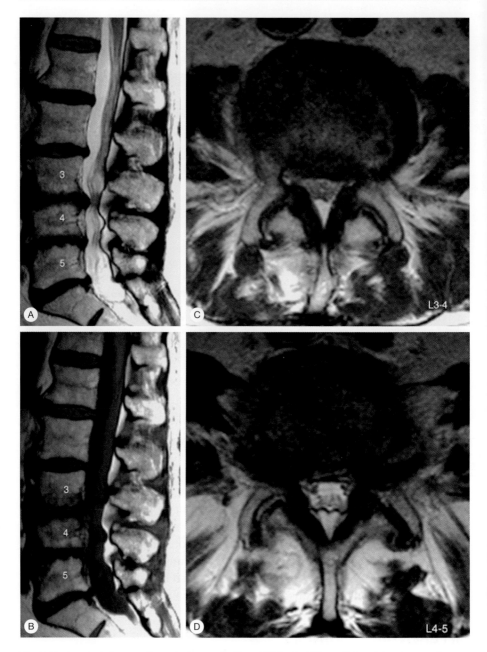

Fig. 14.7   Acquired degenerative spinal stenosis. (A and B) Sagittal T2- and T1-weighted magnetic resonance imaging (MRI) demonstrates severe disc degeneration at L3-L4 and L4-L5, with disc desiccation, disc space narrowing, irregularity of the adjacent vertebral endplates, and posterior bulging discs. The nerve roots of the cauda equine have an undulating or wavy appearance because of the marked constriction at L3-L4. (C and D) On axial T2-weighted MRI, the combination of posterior bulging discs, facet hypertrophy, and thickened ligamenta flava causes severe spinal canal stenosis at L3-L4 and moderate stenosis at L4-L5. Also note severe compromise of the lateral recesses at L3-L4 bilaterally. (From Edelman RR, Hesselink JR, Zlatkin MB, et al., eds. *Clinical Magnetic Resonance Imaging.* 3rd ed. Philadelphia: Saunders; 2006:2228.)

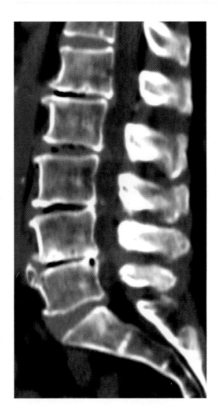

Fig. 14.8 Sagittal computed tomography of a patient with lumbar spinal stenosis that shows disc degeneration with evident loss of disc height, multilevel disc protrusion, along with osteophyte formation, rendering the spinal canal stenotic. (From Biller J, Ferro J. *Handbook of Clinical Neurology*, Vol. 119. Amsterdam: Elsevier; 2014: Fig. 35.1.)

TREATMENT

Spinal stenosis is best treated with a multimodality approach. Physical therapy, including heat modalities and deep sedative massage, combined with nonsteroidal antiinflammatory drugs and skeletal muscle relaxants, is a reasonable starting point. If necessary, caudal or lumbar epidural nerve blocks can be added (Fig. 14.10). Caudal epidural blocks with local anesthetic and steroid are extremely effective in the treatment of spinal stenosis. Underlying sleep disturbance and depression are best treated with a tricyclic antidepressant, such as nortriptyline, which can be started at a single bedtime dose of 25 mg. Recent clinical experience suggests that injection of type A botulinum toxin into the gastrocnemius muscles may also provide symptomatic relief of nocturnal leg cramps associated with lumbar spinal stenosis. If symptoms fail to respond to conservative therapy or neurologic symptoms progress, surgical decompression of the spinal stenosis is indicated.

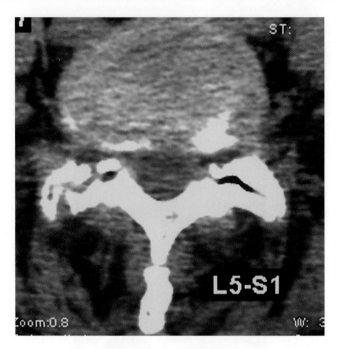

Fig. 14.9   The transaxial computed tomography study at the L5—S1 level shows marked spondyloar-throtic changes involving the L5—S1 facet joints accompanied by anteroposterior diameter and lateral recess stenosis and a focal far lateral right-sided soft herniated disc. (From Quiñones-Hinojosa A. *Schmidek and Sweet Operative Neurosurgical Techniques*. 6th ed. Philadelphia: Saunders; 2016: Management of Far Lateral Lumbar Disc Herniations, Nancy E. Epstien, Fig. 163.16.)

BOX 14.2 ■ Differential Diagnosis of Lumbar Spinal Stenosis

- Herniated cervical disc
- Herniated thoracic disc
- Herniated lumbar disc
- Cervical spinal stenosis
- Thoracic spinal stenosis
- Lumbar spondylosis
- Lumbar spondylolisthesis
- Lumbar facet hypertrophy
- Peripheral vascular disease
- Thombotic ischemia
- Vertebral compression fracture
- Myxedematous claudication
- Inferior vena caval syndrome
- Hip disease
- Sacroiliac disease
- Lower extremity compartment syndromes

(Continued)

- Nerve entrapment syndromes
- Peripheral neuropathy
- Spinal cord tumors
- Metastatic tumors to spine
- Primary tumors of the nerve roots
- Cauda equina tumors
- Perineural fibrosis
- Arachnoiditis
- Restless leg syndrome
- Neurofibromatosis

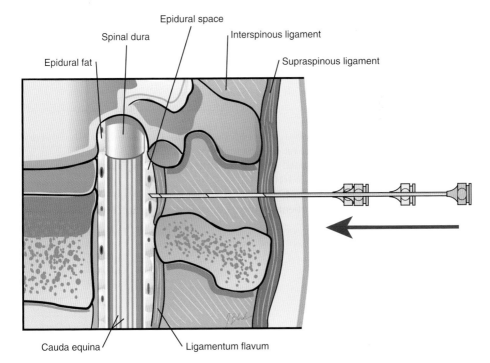

Fig. 14.10 Lumbar epidural block. (From Waldman SD. *Atlas of Interventional Pain Management*. 4th ed. Philadelphia: Saunders; 2015: Fig. 97.8.)

HIGH-YIELD TAKEAWAYS

- The patient's symptomatology is the result of a lifting injury rather than more severe acute trauma, making bony abnormality unlikely.
- The patient's pain is localized in the lower back without radiation into the lower extremities, which makes the diagnosis of lumbar radiculopathy less likely.

(Continued)

- The patient is afebrile, making an infectious etiology unlikely.
- The patient's neurologic examination is normal; specifically, there is no sensory deficit or muscle weakness, and deep tendon reflexes are normal, making a diagnosis of lumbar radiculopathy unlikely.
- There are no bowel or bladder symptoms or pathologic reflexes suggestive of myelopathy.
- The patient has significant sleep disturbance.
- Many pathologic processes can present as low back pain (see Box 9.1).

Suggested Reading

Melancia JL, Francisco AF, Antunes JL. Spinal stenosis. In: Biller J, Ferro JM, eds. *Handbook of Clinical Neurology.* Vol. 1. Philadelphia: Elsevier; 2014:541–549.

Waldman SD. Spinal stenosis. In: Waldman SD, ed. *Atlas of Common Pain Syndromes.* 4th ed. Philadelphia: Elsevier; 2019:324–327.

Maher C, Underwood M, Buchbinder R. Non-specific low back pain. *Lancet.* 2017;389 (10070):736–747.

Meron A, Akuthota V. Spine disorders in older adults. In: Cifu DX, Lew HL, Oh-Park M, eds. *Geriatric Rehabilitation.* 1st ed. Philadelphia: Elsevier; 2018:195–212.

Hartvigsen J, Hancock MJ, Kongsted A, et al. What low back pain is and why we need to pay attention. *Lancet.* 2018;391(10137):2356–2367.

Tan A, Zhou J, Kuo YF, Goodwin JS. Variation among primary care physicians in the use of imaging for older patients with acute low back pain. *J Gen Intern Med.* 2016;31:156–163.

Estella Navarro

A 28-Year-Old Female With Deep Aching in Her Right Low Back and Right Buttock

- Learn the common causes of sacroiliac pain.
- Learn the clinical presentation of sacroiliac pain and dysfunction.
- Learn to distinguish sacroiliac-related pain from lumbar strain and lumbar radiculopathy.
- Learn to identify diseases that might mimic sacroiliac pain.
- Learn the anatomic structures that contribute to sacroiliac pain.
- Develop an understanding of the treatment options for sacroiliac pain.
- Develop an understand ing of the role of physical therapy in the treatment of sacroiliac pain.
- Develop an understanding of the role of interventional pain management in the treatment of sacroiliac pain.

Estella Navarro

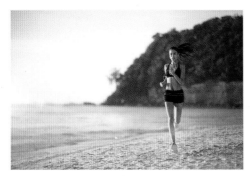

Estella Navarro is a 28-year-old administrative assistant with a chief complaint of, "I hurt my back while running on the beach in Cabo." "Ms. Navarro, when did this pain start?" I asked. "Call me Star," she said. "Well, Doctor," Star began, "I hurt my back while I was on vacation in Cabo with my friend and I just can't seem to get it better. At first, I thought it was my running shoes, so I got new ones, but that didn't help. I tried the usual stuff, changed up my run, ice packs, Advil, but the pain just won't go away. Lately, I have started having the pain even when I'm not exercising. It makes it hard for me to sit for any length of time...it seems like now the pain has kind of settled in my butt...more so on the right...but if I run or sit for very long, the pain spreads to both sides and then it starts to go into the back of my legs."

When I asked Star to show me where the pain was located, she cautiously stood up and pointed to the area over her right sacroiliac joint. She said, "This is where it hurts the worst...but when I jog or sit at my desk for any length of time, the left side starts to hurt and the pain goes down into my butt and the back of my legs...it's kind of like a deep, dull toothache...not sharp or anything...it's kind of hard to pinpoint...oh, and I am having a hard time getting comfortable when I go to bed. And you know, Doctor...it's the strangest thing, it feels like I am always leaning to the right...I try to stand up straight...but I just can't." "Star," I asked, "When the pain goes down the back of your legs, does it ever go past the knees?" She thought for a moment, then slowly shook her head and answered with an emphatic "Never." Star denied any numbness, tingling, or weakness in her legs or feet, but noted that her back muscles "felt tight."

On physical examination, Star was afebrile and normotensive. Star's pulse was a nice, slow 56 and her respirations were 16. Her head, ears, eyes, nose, and throat (HEENT) examination was completely normal, as was her cardiopulmonary examination. Her abdominal examination was also normal. There was no abnormal mass, organomegaly, or peripheral edema. Star's neurologic examination was normal. Specifically, her upper and lower extremity deep tendon reflexes were physiologic, and there was no sensory deficit or weakness in either her arms or legs.

I asked Star to stand up so I could examine her back. She again got up cautiously. I noticed that she was favoring her right leg and had a list to the right. Palpation of the muscles of her lower back revealed tenderness to deep palpation bilaterally. There was also moderate muscle spasm and muscle tightness on the

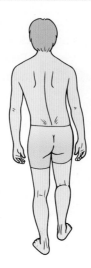

Fig. 15.1 Lateral shifting (lumbar list). (From Norris C. *Managing Sports Injuries*, 4th ed. Churchill Livingstone; 2011: Fig. 13.9C)

right greater than on the left. There were no myofascial trigger points or costovertebral angle tenderness. Star was tender over her sacroiliac joints bilaterally, with the right SI joint being much more tender than the left. I noted decreased flexion of the lumbar spine with a marked exacerbation of pain on extension, right lateral bending, and rotation. The Lasegue test was negative bilaterally. I asked Star to walk and it was obvious that she favored her right leg, had right lateral shifting of the lumbar spine (a list to the right), and walked with an antalgic gait (Fig. 15.1). No pathologic reflexes or clonus were present. I performed the Gaenslen and the Yeoman tests, which were both markedly positive on the right. Pelvic and rectal examination was normal. Star denied bowel and bladder symptoms associated with her pain.

Key Clinical Points—What's Important and What's Not

THE HISTORY

- Chief complaint of "pain in my back that goes into my butt and the back of my legs"
- Sleep disturbance associated with pain
- Recent history of running on an uneven, soft surface (i.e., a sandy beach)
- Lack of significant antecedent trauma to back (e.g., motor vehicle accident, fall)
- Back stiffness and tightness
- Pain is like a deep, dull ache
- Inability to stand up straight

- Feels like she is leaning to the right
- No pain radiation into lower extremities that goes below the knees
- No numbness or weakness of lower extremities
- Symptoms triggered by activity (e.g., jogging or sitting for long periods of time)
- No urinary or fecal incontinence
- No pathologic reflexes

THE PHYSICAL EXAMINATION

- The patient is afebrile
- Lumbar lateral shifting (list) present (see Fig. 15.1)
- Tenderness and spasm of the lumbar paraspinous muscles
- Tenderness of the sacroiliac joints, the right greater than the left
- Normal deep tendon reflexes
- Normal upper and lower extremity motor and sensory examination
- No pathologic reflexes
- No clonus
- Negative Lasegue sign
- Positive Gaenslen and Yeoman tests (Figs. 15.2 and 15.3)

OTHER FINDINGS OF NOTE

- Normal cardiovascular examination
- Normal pulmonary examination
- Normal abdominal examination
- No peripheral edema

 ## What Tests Would You Like to Order?

Given the lack of neurologic findings on Star's physical examination and the lack of significant antecedent trauma, (e.g., motor vehicle accident, fall), I decided to wait on ordering any magnetic resonance imaging (MRIs).

The following tests were ordered:
- Plain radiographs of the lumbar spine
- Plain radiographs of the sacroiliac joints
- Diagnostic block with local anesthetic to further confirm the diagnosis, which immediately relieved almost all of Star's pain (Figs. 15.4 and 15.5)

TEST RESULTS

Star's lumbar spine radiographs were normal, as were her sacroiliac joint x-rays (Fig. 15.6). The good news was that the x-rays did not reveal any occult

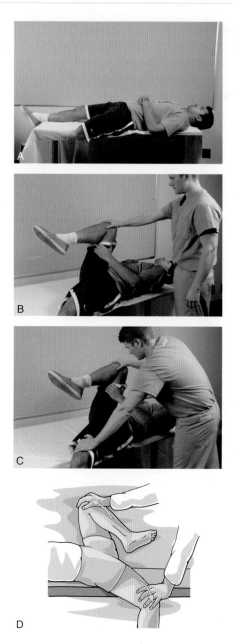

Fig. 15.2 Gaenslen test for sacroiliac joint dysfunction. (A) To perform the Gaenslen test to determine if there is dysfunction of the sacroiliac joint, the patient is placed in the supine position with the painful hip and leg resting on the edge of the examination table. The patient is then asked to move the leg on the painful side so it can hang partially off the examination table. (B) The patient is then asked to flex his or her hip and knee on the nonpainful side to at least 90 degrees and then hold the leg in that position. (C) The patient holds the hip and knee in that position while the examiner stabilizes the pelvis and hip on the nonpainful side by applying firm pressure to the flexed knee and hip. The examiner then applies firm downward pressure to hyperextend the lower extremity that is hanging off the table to put stress on the symptomatic sacroiliac joint. (D) *Arrows* indicate the direction of forces placed on the painful and nonpainful sacroiliac joints. (From Waldman SD. *Physical Diagnosis of Pain: An Atlas of Signs and Symptoms.* 3rd ed. St. Louis: Elsevier; 2016: Figs. 167.1–167.4.)

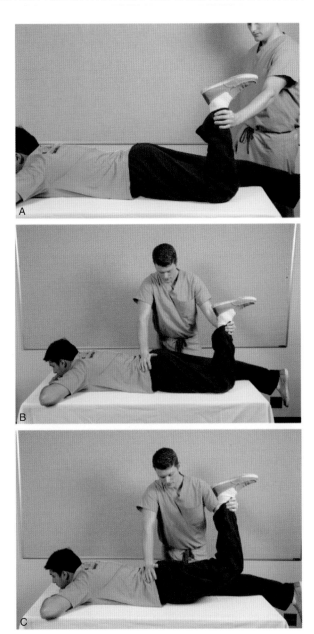

Fig. 15.3 Yeoman test for sacroiliac joint pain. (A) With the patient in prone position, the affected leg is flexed back toward the buttocks to 90 degrees. (B) The examiner then displaces the ipsilateral ilium with firm downward pressure, (C) The examiner then extends the ipsilateral hip. (From Waldman SD. *Physical Diagnosis of Pain: An Atlas of Signs and Symptoms.* 3rd ed. St. Louis: Elsevier; 2016: Figs. 163.1–167.3.)

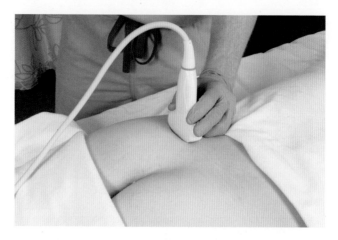

Fig. 15.4 Ultrasound-guided sacroiliac joint injection. Transducer placement. (Courtesy Steven Waldman, MD.)

pathology. Star experienced complete pain relief with a diagnostic ultrasound-guided injection of local anesthetic into the right sacroiliac joint.

Clinical Correlation—Putting It All Together

What is the diagnosis?
- Sacroiliac joint pain

The Science Behind the Diagnosis
ANATOMY OF THE SACROILIAC JOINT

The axial spine rests on the sacrum, a triangular fusion of vertebrae arranged in a kyphotic curve and ending with the attached coccyx in the upper buttock. Iliac wings (innominate bones) attach on either side, forming a bowl with a high back and a shallow front. Three joints result from this union: the pubic symphysis in the anterior midline and the left and right SI joints in the back, and these joints are all susceptible to injury (Fig. 15.7). Multiple ligaments and fascia attach across these joint spaces, limiting motion and providing stability (Figs. 15.8 and 15.9). The hip joints are formed by the femoral heads and the acetabular sockets deep within the innominate bones. The hips create a direct link between the lower extremities and the spine to relay ground reaction forces from weight bearing and motion. A physiologic balance between lumbar lordosis and sacral curvature exists both at rest and in motion. Changes of pelvic tilt and lumbar lordosis occur in the anteroposterior (AP) plane, relying on attached muscles and fascia, but do not have a significant effect on the SI joints owing to a

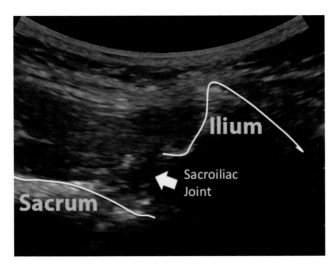

Fig. 15.5 Transverse ultrasound image of the sacroiliac joint. (Courtesy Steven Waldman, MD.)

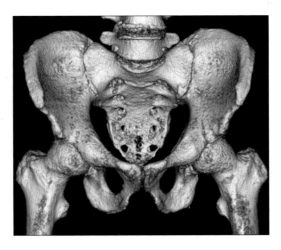

Fig. 15.6 Normal SI joints. (From Polly DW: The sacroiliac joint. *Neurosurg Clin North Am.* 2017;28 (3):301–312, Fig. 1.)

self-bracing mechanism. The sacrum, positioned between the innominate bones, functions as a keystone in an arch, allowing only cephalocaudadal and AP motion. Innervation is varied and extensive owing to the size of this joint, which includes outflow from the anterior and posterior rami of L3-S1.

THE CLINICAL SYNDROME

Pain from the sacroiliac joint commonly occurs when lifting in an awkward position that puts strain on the joint, its supporting ligaments, and soft tissues. The

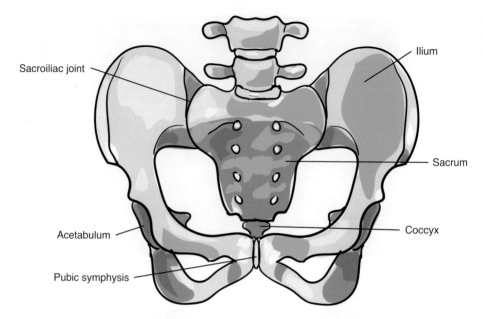

Fig. 15.7 Anatomy of the bony pelvis. (From Waldman SD, Bloch J. *Pain Management*. Philadelphia: Saunders; 2007: Fig. 88.1.)

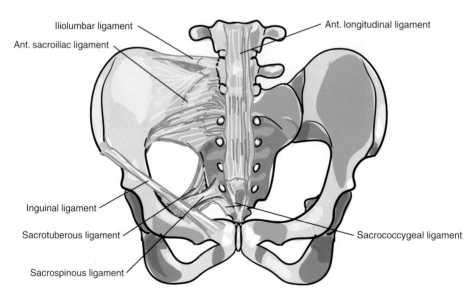

Fig. 15.8 The anterior ligaments of the pelvis. (From Waldman SD, Bloch J. *Pain Management*. Philadelphia: Saunders; 2007: Fig. 88.2.)

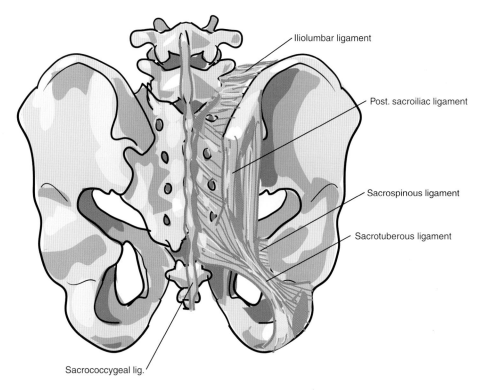

Iliolumbar ligament

Post. sacroiliac ligament

Sacrospinous ligament

Sacrotuberous ligament

Sacrococcygeal lig.

Fig. 15.9 The posterior ligaments of the pelvis. (From Waldman SD, Bloch J. *Pain Management*. Philadelphia: Saunders; 2007: Fig. 88.3.)

sacroiliac joint is also susceptible to the development of arthritis from various conditions that can damage the joint cartilage. Osteoarthritis is the most common form of arthritis that results in sacroiliac joint pain; rheumatoid arthritis and posttraumatic arthritis are also common causes of sacroiliac joint pain. Less-common causes include the collagen vascular diseases, such as ankylosing spondylitis, infection, and Lyme disease (Fig. 15.10). Rarely does the sacroiliac joint become infected (Fig. 15.11). Collagen vascular disease generally manifests as polyarthropathy rather than as monoarthropathy limited to the sacroiliac joint, although sacroiliac pain secondary to ankylosing spondylitis responds exceedingly well to the intraarticular injection technique that will be described later. Occasionally, patients present with iatrogenically induced sacroiliac joint dysfunction resulting from overaggressive bone graft harvesting for spinal fusion.

SIGNS AND SYMPTOMS

Most patients presenting with sacroiliac joint pain secondary to strain or arthritis complain of pain localized around the sacroiliac joint and upper leg that radiates into the

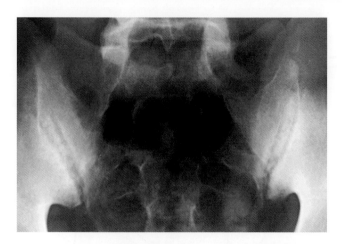

Fig. 15.10   Anteroposterior Ferguson view of the sacroiliac joints in a patient with ankylosing spondylitis, showing bilateral symmetric involvement. Small, succinct erosions involve both sides of the joint, with limited bone repair. (From Waldman SD. *Atlas of Uncommon Pain Syndromes*. 3rd ed. Philadelphia: Saunders; 2014: Fig. 79.2.)

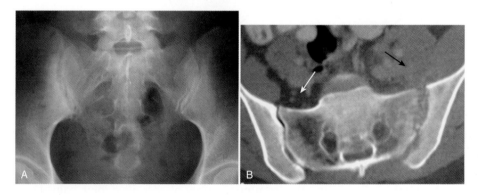

Fig. 15.11   Septic sacrolitis. (A) Anteroposterior radiograph of a patient with right-sided unilateral infective sacroiliitis. There is widening of the joint with loss of the crisp margin of the subchondral bone plate and ill-defined sclerosis. (B) The axial computed tomography scan of a different patient with sacroiliac joint (SIJ) infection shows the same features in the left SIJ. Compare the anterior soft tissue inflammatory mass (*black arrow*) with the normal low-attenuation retroperitoneal fat on the opposite side (*white arrow*). (From Waldman SD, Campbell RSD. Sacroiliac joint pain. In: *Imaging of Pain*. Philadelphia: Elsevier; 2011, Fig. 78.3.)

posterior buttocks and backs of the legs (Fig. 15.12); the pain does not radiate below the knees. Activity makes the pain worse, whereas rest and heat provide some relief. The pain is constant and is characterized as aching; it may interfere with sleep. On physical examination, the affected sacroiliac joint is tender to palpation. The patient often favors the affected leg and lists toward the unaffected side. Spasm of the lumbar paraspinal musculature is often present, as is limited range of motion of the lumbar

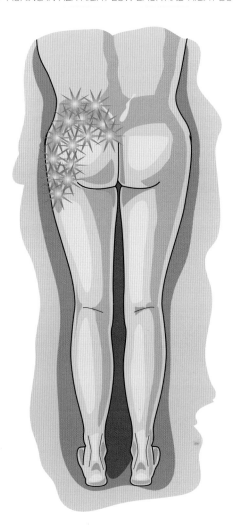

Fig. 15.12   Distribution of pain emanating from the sacroiliac joint. (From Waldman SD, Bloch J. *Pain Management*. Philadelphia: Saunders; 2007: Fig. 88.4.)

spine in the erect position; range of motion improves in the sitting position owing to relaxation of the hamstring muscles. Patients with pain emanating from the sacroiliac joint exhibit a positive pelvic rock test result. This test is performed by placing the examiner's hands on the iliac crests and the thumbs on the anterior superior iliac spines and then forcibly compressing the patient's pelvis toward the midline. A positive test result is indicated by the production of pain around the sacroiliac joint. Other physical examination tests for sacroiliac joint dysfunction include the Yeoman, Gaenslen, Stork, Piedailu, and Van Durson tests (see Figs. 15.2 and 15.3).

TESTING

Plain radiography is indicated in all patients who present with sacroiliac joint pain. Because the sacrum is susceptible to stress fractures and to the development of infection and both primary and secondary tumors, MRI of the distal lumbar spine and sacrum is indicated if the cause of the patient's pain is in question (Fig. 15.13). Computerized tomographic scanning and ultrasound imaging may also provide valuable clinical information (Figs. 15.14 and 15.15). Radionuclide bone scanning should also be considered in such patients to rule out tumor and insufficiency fractures that may be missed on conventional

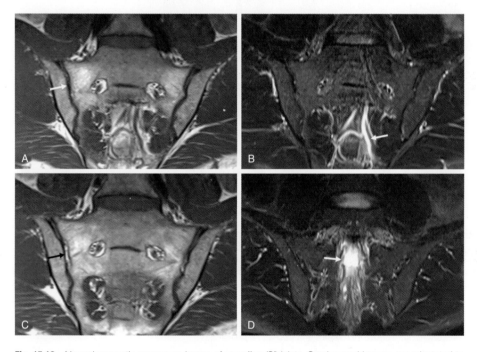

Fig. 15.13   Normal magnetic resonance image of sacroiliac (SI) joints. Semicoronal images are orientated to the long axis of the sacrum and T1-weighted spin echo images (A - anterior slice, C - transitional slice) and STIR images (B - anterior slice, D - posterior slice) are most often acquired. On T1, bone marrow is brighter than muscle because of the higher fat content in bone marrow. The cortical bone appears as a thin dark line marking the joint outline (A - *arrow*). On STIR, the fat signal is suppressed, bone marrow appears darker, and fluid signal is very bright, as seen in presacral veins (B - *arrow*) and cerebrospinal fluid (D - *arrow*). The SI joints extend further anteriorly than sacral vertebral bodies, so anterior parts of the cartilage compartment are visualized on anterior slices (A), along with presacral soft tissues. The transitional slice (C) represents the start of the ligamentous compartment. The transitional slice is best identified on T1-weighted image when fat is seen in the center of the joint (C - *arrow*), representing fat surrounding SI ligaments. Note that on any water-sensitive sequence, small blood vessels are frequently observed as small circular or curvilinear foci of bright signal adjacent to the perimeter of the joint or parallel to ligaments and should not be mistaken for bone marrow or soft tissue inflammation. STIR, short tau inversion recovery. (From Mease P, Khan M. *Axial Spondyloarthritis*. St. Louis: Elsevier; 2020: Fig. 10.5.)

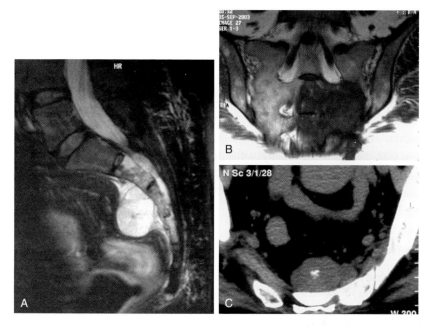

Fig. 15.14   Sacral chordoma. Sagittal, fast spin-echo, T2-weighted (A) and axial T1-weighted (B) magnetic resonance images show a large soft tissue mass arising from the sacrum with bony destruction. The bulk of the tumor is presacral. Axial computed tomography scan (C) demonstrates bony involvement of the left half of the sacrum by a large midline presacral mass with calcification. (From Edelman RR, Hesselink JR, Zlatkin MB, et al., eds. *Clinical Magnetic Resonance Imaging.* 3rd ed. Philadelphia: Saunders; 2006:2333.)

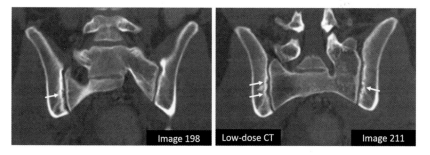

Fig. 15.15   Low-dose computed tomography (LD-CT) confirms the presence of sacroiliitis in a young adult male. These 1.5-mm thick coronal images were reconstructed at 1-mm increments. Small subchondral erosions (*arrows*) in the right ilium were seen on many of the images. However, definite erosion of the left ilium was seen only on a single coronal slice. LD-CT provides excellent visualization of structural damage in the sacroiliac (SI) joints regardless of the orientation of the articular surface and without superimposition of bony structures and overlying bowel. SI joint LD-CT can be consistently performed with radiation exposure of less than 1 mSv, which is in the same exposure range as radiography for the SI joints with oblique views and with less radiation exposure than radiographs in some larger patients. (From Mease P, Khan M. *Axial Spondyloarthritis.* St. Louis: Elsevier; 2020: Fig. 10.4.)

radiographs. Based on the patient's clinical presentation, additional testing may be warranted, including a complete blood count, erythrocyte sedimentation rate, human leukocyte antigen (HLA)-B27 screening, antinuclear antibody testing, and automated blood chemistry.

DIFFERENTIAL DIAGNOSIS

Pain emanating from the sacroiliac joint can be confused with low back strain; lumbar bursitis; lumbar fibromyositis; piriformis syndrome; ankylosing spondylitis; inflammatory arthritis; and disorders of the lumbar spinal cord, roots, plexus, and nerves (Box 15.1). Remember, sacroiliac pain may coexist with other causes of low back pain (Box 15.2).

TREATMENT

Sacroiliac joint pain is best treated with a multimodality approach (Box 15.3). Initial treatment of the pain and functional disability of sacroiliac joint pain includes a combination of nonsteroidal antiinflammatory drugs or cyclooxygenase-2 inhibitors and physical therapy. The local application of heat and cold may also be beneficial. For patients who do not respond to these treatment modalities, injection with local anesthetic and a steroid is a reasonable next step. Injection of the sacroiliac joint is carried out by placing the patient in the supine position and preparing the skin overlying the affected sacroiliac joint space with antiseptic solution. A sterile syringe containing 4 mL of 0.25% preservative-free bupivacaine and 40 mg methylprednisolone is attached to a

---

BOX 15.1 ■ Common Causes of Sacroiliac Joint-Related Pain

- Psoriatic arthritis
- Reiter's syndrome
- Septic arthritis
- Ulcerative colitis
- Crohn's disease
- Synovitis-acne-pustulosis hyperostosis-osteomyelitis (SAPHO) syndrome
- Seronegative arthropathies, including ankylosing spondylitis
- Tuberculosis
- Intestinal bypass-induced arthritis
- Sarcoidosis
- Whipple's disease
- Brucellosis
- Hyperparathyroidism

BOX 15.2 ■ Differential Diagnosis of Low Back Pain

- Mechanical etiology
- Degenerative disc disease
- Facet arthropathy
- Spinal stenosis
- Spondylolisthesis
- Spondylolysis
- Traumatic transverse process fracture
  - Kyphosis
  - Scoliosis
  - Congenital abnormalities of the vertebra, e.g. transitional vertebra, trefoil canal

Nonmechanical Etiology
- Primary neoplasm
- Metastatic disease
- Osteomyelitis
- Multiple myeloma
- Paget disease of bone
- Myofascial pain
- Discitis
- Epidural abscess
- Paraspinal abscess
- Retroperitoneal tumors
- Spinal cord tumors
- Lymphoma
- Leukemia
- Herpes zoster
- Ankylosing spondylitis
- Reiter syndrome
- Psoriatic arthritis
- Scheuermann's disease

Visceral Disease
- Pancreatitis
- Renal calculi
- Ureteral calculi
- Chloecystitis
- Posterior penetrating gastric ulcer
- Idiopathic

25-gauge needle using strict aseptic technique. The posterior superior spine of the ilium is identified. At this point, the needle is carefully advanced through the skin and subcutaneous tissues at a 45-degree angle toward the affected sacroiliac joint. If bone is encountered, the needle is withdrawn into the subcutaneous tissues and is redirected superiorly and slightly more laterally. After the joint space is entered, the contents of the syringe are gently injected. Little resistance to

> ### BOX 15.3 ■ Treatment Modalities For Sacroiliac Pain
>
> **Physical Modalities**
> - Physical therapy
> - Local heat
> - Deep sedative massage
> - Ice rubs
>
> **Medication Management**
> - Simple analgesics
> - Nonsteroidal antiinflammatory agents
> - Cyclooxygenase-2 inhibitors
>
> **TENS unit**
> *Manipulative therapy*
> **Interventional Pain Management**
> - Intraarticular sacroiliac joint injections

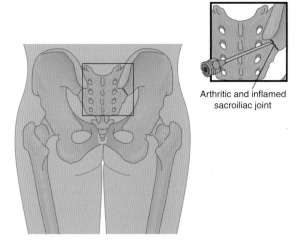

Arthritic and inflamed
sacroiliac joint

Fig. 15.16   Correct needle placement for injection of the sacroiliac joint. (From Waldman SD. *Atlas of Pain Management Injection Techniques*. Philadelphia: Saunders; 2000.)

injection should be felt. If resistance is encountered, the needle is probably in a ligament and should be advanced slightly into the joint space until the injection can proceed without significant resistance. The needle is then removed, and a sterile pressure dressing and ice pack are applied to the injection site. The use of fluoroscopy, computed tomography, and ultrasound guidance may be required in patients in whom the anatomic landmarks are difficult to identify (see Figs. 15.5, 15.16, and 15.17). Physical modalities, including local heat and gentle

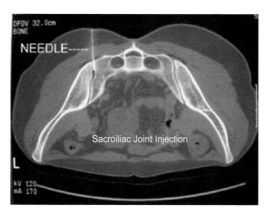

Fig. 15.17 Computed tomography (CT) images of sacroiliac joint injection. Courtesy Steven D. Waldman.

BOX 15.4 ■ Red Flags In Patients Suffering From Sacroiliac Pain

- History of significant trauma
- Nonmechanical back pain
- Past history of cancer
- Unexplained fever
- Unexplained weight loss or inanition
- Bony abnormality
- Abnormal neurologic examination
- Altered sensorium
- Presence of pathologic reflexes
- Alterations of gait

---

range-of-motion exercises, should be introduced several days after the patient undergoes injection for sacroiliac pain. Vigorous exercises should be avoided, because they will exacerbate the patient's symptoms.

HIGH-YIELD TAKEAWAYS

- The patient's symptomatology is the result of a lifting injury rather than more severe acute trauma, making bony abnormality unlikely.
- The patient's pain is localized in the lower back without radiation into the lower extremities, which makes the diagnosis of lumbar radiculopathy less likely.
- The patient is afebrile, making an infectious etiology unlikely.

(Continued)

BOX 15.5 ■ Diseases That May Mimic Sacroiliac Joint Dysfunction

- Lumbar disc disease
- Primary tumors of the bony pelvis
- Primary tumors of the nerves of the pelvis
- Metastatic tumors to the region
- Infection
- Ankylosing spondylitis
- Spondyloarthropathy
- Hip joint pathology
- Superior cluneal nerve entrapment
- Tendonitis of the hip and pelvis
- Bursitis of the hip and pelvis
- Snapping hip syndrome
- Iliotibial band syndrome
- Lumbosacral facet syndrome
- Lumbosacral radiculopathy
- Piriformis syndrome
- Sacroiliac joint infection
- Trochanteric bursitis

- The patient's neurologic examination is normal; specifically, there is no sensory deficit or muscle weakness and deep tendon reflexes are normal, making a diagnosis of lumbar radiculopathy unlikely.
- There are no bowel or bladder symptoms or pathologic reflexes suggestive of myelopathy.
- The patient has significant sleep disturbance.
- Many pathologic processes can present as low back pain (see Boxes 15.1—15.5).

Suggested Reading

Booth J, Morris S. The sacroiliac joint—victim or culprit. *Best Practice & Research Clinical Rheumatology*. 2019;33(1):88—101.

Isaac Z, Brassil ME: Sacroiliac joint dysfunction. In: Frontera WR, Silver JK, Rizzo TD, eds. *Essentials of Physical Medicine and Rehabilitation*. 4th ed. Elsevier: Philadelphia; 2020:284—290.

Emery CA, Pasanen K. Current trends in sport injury prevention. *Best Practice & Research Clinical Rheumatology*. 2019;33(1):3—15.

Maher C, Underwood M, Buchbinder R. Non-specific low back pain. *Lancet*. 2017;389 (10070):736—747.

Hartvigsen J, Hancock MJ, Kongsted A, et al. What low back pain is and why we need to pay attention. *Lancet*. 2018;391(10137):2356—2367.

Qaseem A, Wilt TJ, McLean RM, Forciea MA. Noninvasive treatments for acute, sub-acute, and chronic low back pain: a clinical practice guideline from the American College of Physicians. *Ann Intern Med*. 2017;166(7):514–530.

Qaseem A, Wilt TJ, McLean RM, Forciea MA. Noninvasive treatments for acute, sub-acute, and chronic low back pain: a clinical practice guideline from the American College of Physicians. *Ann Intern Med*. 2017;166(7):514–530.

Tan A, Zhou J, Kuo YF, Goodwin JS. Variation among primary care physicians in the use of imaging for older patients with acute low back pain. *J Gen Intern Med*. 2016;31:156–163.

INDEX

Page numbers followed by 'f' indicate figures, 't' indicate tables, 'b' indicate boxes.

)